Folk Dances of Jamaica:
An Insight

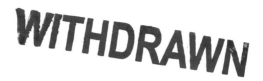

Folk Dances of Jamaica: An Insight

A study of five folk dances of Jamaica with regard to the origins, history, development, contemporary setting and dance technique of each

Hilary S. Carty

Dance Books
Cecil Court   London

First published in 1988 by Dance Books Ltd.,
9 Cecil Court, London WC2N 4EZ.

© 1988 Hilary S. Carty

Distributed in the United States of America
by Princeton Book Co., P.O. Box 57,
Pennington, N.J. 08534.

British Library Cataloguing in Publication Data
Carty, Hilary S.
   Folk dances of Jamaica: an insight, a study of five
   dances of Jamaica with regard to the origins, history,
   development, contemporary setting and dance
   technique of each.
   1. Jamaican folk dancing
   I. Title
   793.3'197292
   ISBN 1-85273-007-2

Design and production in association with
Book Production Consultants, 47 Norfolk St., Cambridge
Typeset by Goodfellow and Egan, Cambridge
Printed by Oxford University Press

Acknowledgements

I wish to thank all who helped to make my year in Jamaica a profitable and enjoyable one, particularly Leila Spence, Neville Spence, Veronica Lovindeer, Rahshema Lovindeer, Sarah Bailey-Coke and Anthony Johnson.

Special thanks for the encouragement and assistance of: Mrs Sheila Barnett, Director, Jamaica School of Dance; Mr Bert Rose, Jamaica School of Dance; Mr Barry Moncrieffe, Jamaica School of Dance; Mrs Barbara Requa, Jamaica School of Dance; Miss Cheryl Ryman, African Caribbean Institute of Jamaica.

To the 1983/84 students of the Jamaica School of Dance I extend much gratitude for welcoming me into the group and securing my place there. My gratitude also to Joe Robinson and Evelyn Toppin for their encouragement, support and assistance throughout the year.

For all the time and effort expended in helping me to realise my goals I wish to thank Earle Robinson M.B.E., 'H' Patten for the beautiful illustrations and Wendy Francis for the endless hours spent at the typewriter.

To all those unmentioned who have helped along the way: Thank you.

CONTENTS

Preface

Linked as they are to our historical and social development and to rituals, religious and secular, traditional dances are a significant component of the Jamaican cultural experience. These traditional forms, which were clearly identifiable by the nineteenth century, are the result of the interaction of Africa and Europe (the British).

Hilary Carty has studied, researched and practised a number of traditional core types during a year spent in Jamaica at such institutions as the Jamaica School of Dance and the African Caribbean Institute of Jamaica. She also devoted time to field trips and the study of selected dances in their functional environment. In this book Miss Carty has combined background information and content of five core types. The selection is representative of religious expression, funerary rites and social dances both European derived (Quadrille) and Creolised (Bruckin's). The final chapter, 'Abstraction: Towards a Technique', presents basic features of the Jamaican traditional dances and includes suggestions for further development in such a way as to inspire teachers, performers and community leaders who are involved with the Black Dance experience.

The material in this book is not intended for beginners. The codification of movement and steps demands a basic knowledge of dance. The text is intended for dancers and teachers of dance who wish to further the knowledge and skills learned through contact sources such as workshops and seminars or through brief visits to the Caribbean.

Of particular value are the 'How To Do' sections with their detailed illustrations, information and drawings prepared by 'H' Patten, a dancer, artist and teacher. 'H's knowledge of Caribbean dance has been reinforced through visits to Jamaica, Trinidad and Tobago. These sections focus on such technical aspects of Caribbean dance as stance, body movements and steps.

The writer has chosen to emphasise common basic elements of what might become a system of training. She has also included instructions concerning the performing of specific Jamaican dances – Kumina, Dinkie Minie, Quadrille, Bruckin's and Revival.

Sheila Barnett, M. A.
Director, Jamaica School of Dance
October 1986

Introduction

The first European visit to Jamaica was made by Christopher Columbus, in 1494. Like most other Caribbean islands, its development since then has involved three major factors: Occupation – the Caribbean islands were occupied by adventurers from all over Europe, in the case of Jamaica these being predominantly British; Importation – African slaves were imported into the islands to work the sugar plantations, which were the major source of income, until the late eighteenth century; Colonisation – as a result of the European occupation the majority of the islands in the Caribbean basin were colonised and remained under foreign rule until the twentieth century. Some islands, e.g. Martinique and Guadeloupe, are colonised even today. Jamaica gained its independence from Britain in 1962. These three factors, occupation, importation and colonisation, have left a considerable mark on the Jamaica of today, in terms of the national outlook, governmental procedures and even the population of the island – along with the English who settled and the Africans who were brought to Jamaica came also the Spanish, Welsh, Scottish, Indians and Chinese. Hence, Jamaica today is the product of a combination of sources. Over the centuries, Jamaicans have selected and merged items from each cultural influence, bringing them together under one cultural roof, to be housed in the Jamaican way of life. Even with this combination of sources, however, the two major cultural influences on Jamaica can be pin-pointed as African and British, as these two cultures were most crucial to the make-up and growth of the country.

In 1494 the island was captured by Christopher Columbus in the name of King Ferdinand and Queen Isabella of Spain and the Spanish ruled the island until 1665 when it was captured by British soldiers. The British rulers, wishing to place a firm hold on the island, drew their citizens there with land grants and other financial enticements. Others went as indentured labourers working for a specific length of time and, as an alternative to a prison sentence in England, many convicts were sent to Jamaica to serve their time. At first the majority were reluctant to travel to the Caribbean islands, which were largely uncultivated and had a decidedly hot climate, but in a relatively short space of time the popularity of the West Indies grew, largely due to the introduction and cultivation of sugar plantations, the lucrative income from which enabled many to return home rich.

Historians cite the introduction of sugar as the most influential factor in the growth and development of Jamaica. Firstly, with the increased world-wide demand for sugar in preference to honey for sweetening tea and coffee, its cultivation became a vital asset to the island's capturers:

> The Spaniards, and after them adventurers of all nations, came to the Indies seeking rich mines of gold and silver, but as they were to discover in time, the real wealth of the Indies was the wide fields of sugar cane. In their 18th century hey-day the 'sugar colonies' as the islands came to

be called were the most valuable possession of any empire, fiercely fought over in every war that broke out in Europe and as fiercely bargained for at every peace conference.[1]

Secondly, the plantations directly affected the population content of Jamaica. Had other crops proved lucrative, the enormous increase in slave trading, which had in fact begun during Spanish rule, might not have been necessary. But, as well as the need for vast areas of land, sugar cultivation required a large, hard-working labour force. Thus, sugar and slavery went hand in hand. The land was readily available, much of it owned by a few wealthy planters. The labour force, however, was not so easy to come by. There were some Europeans on the island fit to work the plantations but as they required payment their labour proved too expensive and resulted in a reduction in the profits. Nor were there really enough indentured labourers to cope with the work load. The British solution to this problem was therefore to continue the practice begun by the Spaniards. Under the Treaty of Utrecht (1713), Britain took over from France the 'Asiento', the contract to distribute African slaves to the Spanish colonies. So although the slaves were originally brought in to work the sugar plantations, the slave trade to Jamaica increased 'tenfold. Alongside Barbados and the other English speaking Caribbean Islands, Jamaica remained a distribution centre for slaves until 1807 when the practice was made illegal'.[2]

It must be noted, however, 'that both the British masters and their slaves, who were later to come in huge numbers [to Jamaica], were total strangers to the land upon which they were destined to build a completely new society. The vast majority of the people who were to mould this society came against their will. This was true not only of the slaves, but the large number of Irish, Welsh, Scottish and English, who, coming originally as indentured servants and later under the pressure of economic deprivation, were as much the victims of the capitalist exploiters of England as were the bewildered tribesmen of Africa whose labour they were to supervise.'[3]

However, the major difference in situation was that while the British came 'to supervise' and by retaining control could dictate their own movements, the Africans were bought and brought into the country with no control over their lives. Subordinates from the very outset, they were denied all rights: individual rights, cultural rights, the right to live as they wished. Regarded as empty vessels, they had nothing to offer but their labour. Their days, nights and all activities were planned for them and, like children, they were allowed recreation only according to the rules and whims of their 'parents', the British.

The story of the African slave brought into the West Indies is a peculiar one of inhumane treatment of one race by another. Taken from his natural surroundings, the slave was deliberately separated from his kin and tribesmen, and thus all links with his past life were broken. Forced to work and mix with others who, more often than not, spoke a different language, he was forced to find a new means of communication. Placed in an alien environment and made to perform alien functions as part of his daily timetable, he was forced to adopt a whole new lifestyle. Life on the plantation was busy and arduous; slaves were made to work long hours and, as production and profit were the master's first concern, the welfare of the slave was not always regarded. Brutal treatment of slaves was common practice. The greatest abuse, however, was that he was given no real control over his being or his actions. The slave's life was determined by his role and duties on the plantation. Work duties naturally dictated recreational hours; both were dictated by the master. It was the master who gave permission for social activities to take place, the master who banned or encouraged certain African religious practices and who inadvertently played a vital part in the continuation and development of African dance and social practices.

With so much of his culture forbidden him, the African slave, used to a tradition of dance, drumming and song as a means of worship and indeed an intrinsic part of life itself, was forced to continue these practices in the evenings or as much as his work schedule would allow. Getting together in groups, they practised their social/religious customs of rituals, ancestor worship and burial rites until the master, seeing how frenzied they would become, forbade them to continue these practices. The drum was thought dangerous as it was believed to incite the slaves to rebellion and so the drum was banned also. But the Africans showed their creativity by fashioning instruments from available local materials: much use was made of the calabash, for shakas, and to make the body of the 'benta' (a long string instrument used in Dinkie Minie and Gerreh); drums were fashioned from kerosene tins, and numerous hand percussion instruments were made from household items like small tins and graters. Knives and forks were often used to hit or scrape the instruments. Even while these instruments were being made, however, some slaves continued to play the African drum in secret as it formed a central part of their worship (see Chapter One: Kumina). Thus certain drum patterns, 'breaks' (a short musical interruption to the melody, usually played on the female drum), and the drum-making procedure were secretly passed on to each new generation. Kumina for example, the most 'African' of Jamaican folk dances, is described by Braithwaite as:

> . . . the living fragment of an African (mainly kongo) religion in the Caribbean/Jamaica. It is a fragment because the slave/plantation system did not allow more than fragments: the visible public aspects of the incoming (so-called deracinated) Africans were, in the instinctive interests of control, suppressed; the social language, the social hierarchies, the specialists, the public customary observances, and therefore the officials of symbol, regalia and publicly expressed ritual, link and memory, were destroyed. Therefore African culture in the slave world, to survive . . . had to submerge itself, had to lose much of its public visibility; had, as it submerged, to accept losses, to adapt; miraculously, creatively did this; persisted and survived.[4]

Thus evidently, in cases of African-derived dances like Kumina, the white plantocracy mainly affected the development of the ritual by restricting its time of practice, thus curbing some of its fervour. The nature and content of the customs, however, remained, for the most part, intact.

In the case of European-derived dance forms, the retentions are much less evident. To a certain extent it is correct to say that the most striking and lasting of the two cultural influences (African/European) is the African contribution. This is evident in terms of both content and performance practices. (Note the African influence on Kumina, Revival, Dinkie Minie and Bruckin's.) On the European side, we see evidence of strong retentions in Jonkonnu, a colourful masquerade of characters (also known in the African tradition), but mainly in the Quadrille. Three factors can help to pin-point the reason for the apparent weakness of the European influence. Firstly, in chronological terms, the European connection was rather late in coming: while African rituals had been incorporated into the plantation society since its inception, the Quadrille, the first European dance really to take shape in Jamaica, was not introduced into society there until the eighteenth century, when the dance was popular also in Europe. Cheryl Ryman suggests that one reason for this is that there was no real 'community' of Europeans in Jamaica before this time and thus social and religious communal practices had not yet taken any definite shape or form.[5] Secondly, the physical number of Europeans could in no way match that of the Africans. With the system of Absenteeism, whereby plantation owners lived abroad and left the everyday running of the plantation to overseers, the European contingent could not but be limited. Thirdly, the folk traditions of Jamaica, like those of most countries, are mainly continued within the communities of the lower strata of society and, in Jamaica, these are mainly of African descent. It is quite natural, therefore, that they retain mainly African traits.

The European traditions were mainly passed on through social circumstances. The Africans observed the European stance, behaviour and dance styles at the 'Plantation Revelries', which were the major social and recreational activities of the Europeans. On these occasions the house slaves were able to observe and copy the styles and stance of their masters. These were later passed on to the field slaves who, in turn, adopted and adapted the movements and postures to fit their own style of dance. This provoked the evolution of forms such as Bruckin's and the Camp Style Quadrille, which are indigenous Jamaican dance forms revealing a blend of African and European traditions. It must be noted, however, that opportunities for even observing European behaviour on a social level were few and these restricted only to house slaves. This also had a direct effect on the level and quantity of European customs and styles that could be passed on.

For the slaves themselves the major source of organised (i.e. by the master) social activity were the holiday feasts such as Easter, Christmas and Crop-Over. These

> . . . gave relief from the tedium and severity of slavery, from the constant onslaught on the self-dignity and pride of the slave. On this day they were allowed to dress in all their finery and assume new names. A certain degree of familiarity with the masters was permitted.

Thirdly, the feast day provided the slave with an outlet from pent-up aggressions and hostilities against the masters. Tension could be released through the energetic and vigorous dances such as Camp Style Quadrille, Jonkonnu, an Xmas-time masquerade, and others. Jonkonnu, like Bruckin's, includes a section for 'set' rivalry. Here, groups dressed in Red or Blue and tried to out-dance each other. This was a subtle method of re-directing the anger against the master by challenging their 'set' rival. Some of the aggression could be directed at the master, but again, subtly through miming and caricaturing of the whites and the satire of the songs sung on these occasions.[6]

It was on feast days such as these that the true merging of styles took shape as the constant copying of movements led to an eventual adoption of the very same movements that were being mimicked. Thus the true Jamaican culture began. The true Jamaican culture must and can only refer to that which evolved in Jamaica, under Jamaican influences. The African and European practices, in their natural context, underwent particular changes, but it is the adaptions that evolved in Jamaica that are of interest here. The Jamaican dimension is in fact a 'creolisation' of influences and forms – the blending together of alien customs, beliefs and practices to arrive at a version unique to its creators. Creolisation, states Nettleford, refers to the process of renewal and growth that marks the new order of men and women who came originally from different Old World cultures and met, in conflict or otherwise, on foreign soil.[7]

'New order' had to evolve because the circumstances and lifestyles of the men and women from Africa and Europe had changed. The second generation of both masters and slaves on the island were Jamaican-born. What did they, cut off from the original source, create as culture? As has been stated, the Europeans were better able to keep up with their homelands through frequent visits, and it is to the Jamaican-born slaves that we must look for the truest creolisation process, which, with its necessity for borrowing, selecting and adapting, is the most striking feature of the Jamaican culture. This creolisation is reflected in the merging of languages: the slaves never quite mastered the English of their masters but adapted it to create their own Patois. It is reflected in the instruments used to accompany their dances: they were forbidden to use the drums of Africa but this did not stop them from creating their own instruments and rhythms from any available material. It is also reflected in the dances themselves: the Africans never perfected the European style Quadrille but still they danced it, with African features such as the flexed foot, tilted body, and use of broken lines. Most significant in this area, therefore, are folk forms such as Bruckin's and the religious practices of the Revivalist cults. These forms, as discussed in their respective chapters, reveal the natural fibres of Jamaican culture. Both post-emancipation forms, their significance lies in their departure from a direct African or European source. They are syncretisms, yes, but in every way as indigenous to Jamaica as the national Doctor Bird.

The folk forms of Jamaica are to be found all over the island, even while regional differences and preferences for particular forms exist. This is reflective of the lives and customs of the peoples that settled in each parish. Thus the term 'land of contrasts', as Jamaica is often described in the tourist brochures, is indeed correct. Underlying these contrasts, however, in terms of style, motivation and performance practices, is a consistency of form. This has been made possible because Jamaica, though influenced by many, has somewhat miraculously derived a culture and style of its own. The process of selection is now complete and the national motto 'Out of Many One People' is pertinent to the customs and practices of that people also: 'Out of Many: One Culture'.

This study has been undertaken after a year of research into the nature and practice of the Jamaican folk dance forms. As such, it does not presume to cover the whole sector but is a collation and summary of information gleaned so far on five of the dance forms. The writer intends to expand this research to clarify and enrich her knowledge further. The aim of this study is to define and describe some core types of the Jamaican folk forms. By providing a brief history of each form the dances will be placed in context in terms of origin, main influences, major characteristics and usage today. The dances themselves will then be discussed in technical terms of characteristic steps, body stance and how to perform each step. It is hoped that by giving detailed descriptions of the steps, the reader will receive a clearer and more functional insight into the folk dances of Jamaica. These dances have been categorised as follows:

1. African-derived, i.e. revealing the most African retentions.
2. European-derived, i.e. revealing the most European retentions.
3. Indigenous creolised, i.e. revealing the particular Jamaican trait of adoption, adaption and eventual creolisation.
4. 'Abstraction: Towards a Technique' in Chapter Four shows ways in which the same folk dances can be manipulated to create new and exciting movements towards the development of a modern folk technique and dance style. While it is important to maintain the folk dances in their original form, the writer also sees a need for development of these forms in a contemporary idiom, to encourage growth and appreciation of these forms by contemporary folk.

The folk dances of Jamaica are central in its history and development.

Dance has done much more than preserve the movement expressions of our people, it is both catalyst and agent . . . as catalyst it generates and continues to give meaning to activities like the preparation of fufu (food of African origin) and as agent, it remains the single most important vehicle through which to recall the past and reveal the essence of Jamaican culture.[8]

1. Black (1983), p. 68.
2. Norris (1962), p. 2.
3. Patterson (1973), p. 9.
4. Braithwaite, C.K., 'Kumina: The Spirit of African Survival in Jamaica'. *Jamaica Journal* (1949), No. 42, p. 46.
5. Ryman, C., 'Caribbean Literature', Jamaica School of Dance, 1984.
6. Patterson, *op. cit.*, p. 248
7. Nettleford (1974).
8. Ryman, C., 'The Jamaican Heritage in Dance'. *Jamaica Journal* (1980), No. 44, p. 3.

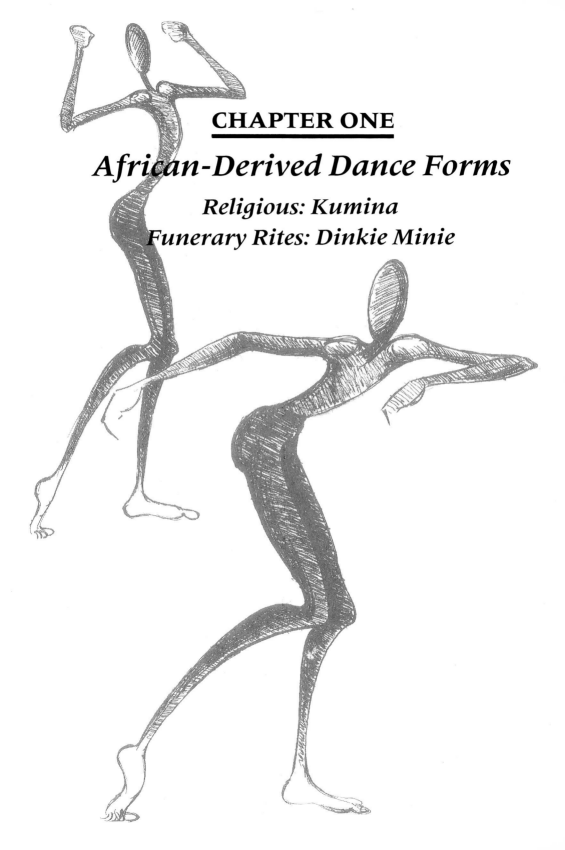

CHAPTER ONE

African-Derived Dance Forms

Religious: Kumina
Funerary Rites: Dinkie Minie

Kumina

Kumina is a ritual said to have originated in the Congo region of West Africa. As such it reveals the strongest African retentions of all the Jamaican folk dances. Professor Rex Nettleford states that this can be traced in three ways.

Firstly, the motions and positions used in the dance are exclusively African in style and stance, incorporating a version of what has now been termed the 'Congo Step'. Secondly, in terms of linguistics, authentic African words spoken by the dancers can be distinguished at Kumina rituals. These words, as with much of the Kumina tradition, have been passed on verbally from generation to generation. Thirdly, the paraphernalia or mediums used at a ritual – e.g. rum, water and animal sacrifice – have direct links with African ritualistic practices. Also, the music created in Kumina rituals has been traced back to Africa and similarities of form and content have been noted even today.[1]

The authenticity of Kumina's Congolese roots can further be proved in that the practitioners of Kumina in Jamaica, mainly from St Thomas, St Mary and West Kingston, claim never to have been slaves. If this is so, then they are evidently descendants of the large number of Congolese men and women brought into the island after 1807 when the slave trade was abolished. These Africans came to Jamaica as freemen and indentured labourers.[2] It would therefore follow that, as freemen, they were not as strongly influenced by the European culture as the captive slave and could openly continue their own social, religious and ritualistic practices. A large settlement of Kumina dancers can also be found in Maroon Town, which indeed remained an independent community of black Africans and descendants throughout the British rule, the Maroons having successfully defended themselves from British attacks until they were allowed self-rule. Kumina is generally found among peoples from the lower strata of society who, lacking the 'sophistication' of external influences, stick closer to their roots – in this case West African.

Kumina practitioners believe in the existence of three ranks of spirits; Sky, Earth, and Ancestral. The Sky spirits, carry the highest rank and have the strongest powers. Second in rank are the Earth spirits, who may appear by 'entering' the body of a practitioner. The Ancestral spirits are third in line in terms of rank, but first in usage: the Sky and Earth spirits are said to have a much wider hemisphere in which to work and, as such, are least accessible to individuals. Thus the Ancestral spirits are more frequently called upon to work for their descendants. The Kumina ritual is performed in celebration; of a birth, marriage, engagement, political or social success etc. It may also be performed at a wake ceremony as part of the Set-Up and Ninth-Night activities (see Chapter One: Dinkie Minie). Kumina may even be used for evil purposes, to do someone ill, wish them bad luck, or make them physically sick. All this is possible because the Kumina ritual focuses on the calling of Ancestral spirits, who, having shared our mortality, share also our desires for justice and revenge. Patterson, in *The Sociology of Slavery* (1973: p. 199) also suggests that homage was paid to the Ancestral spirits because Africans were more afraid of their own ancestors than of the Gods.

Barry Moncrieffe, in a lecture on Traditional Folk Forms, stated that a Kumina ritual usually begins at sundown and may well last to sun-up the next day. The ritual takes place in the round and a central pole decked in colours is essential to the ceremony: the colours of the pole and also the colours of the participants' costumes tell the occasion for the ritual. The dance is led by a Kumina King or Queen who is usually the best dancer and the member most versed in the customs and practices of Kumina rituals. He or she must also have full knowledge of the folk songs and drum rhythms, as these are two of the mediums through which the spirits are called. Other mediums through which the spirits may travel include White Rum (alcohol is always intrinsic to rituals in Jamaica); sugar; cream-soda; candles; water (carried on the head to 'catch the spirit'); coconut (said to have the power to prevent harm); and blood from a goat or fowl.[3] Animal sacrifice is a common factor of rituals worldwide. In Jamaica the blood of the animal is mixed with White Rum and 'fed' to the spirits through spraying.

Two general types of song are sung at Kumina rituals: 'Bailo' (at the more public, less sacred form of Kumina at which time songs are sung mainly in Jamaican dialect) and 'Country' (the more African and serious form, at which time possession usually occurs).[4] Antiphony (call and response pattern), a common feature of African tradition, is used in Kumina. Also African is the practice of the drum leading the dance and, indeed, the ritual, which *is* a dance. Thus it is considered a position of honour to be a drummer at a Kumina ritual.

Two types of drum, made from hollow cedar logs, are used for Kumina. The Kbandu is the male drum, the head of which is made from the skin of a ewe. In the drum-making ritual, the stretched skin is repeatedly sprayed with White Rum until the required pitch is achieved. The White Rum is said to help cure the skin and thus the practice of spraying the head of the drum with rum before a ceremony (libation) is functional as well as spiritual. The female drum, the Playing Cast, is the leading instrument in Kumina and has a higher tone than the Kbandu. It is the one that 'speaks', directing the dancers through the motions and the 'breaks'. This is reflective of the African tradition which is both Matriarchal and Matrilineal.[5] While both drums are played with the hand and fingers, the tone of the Kbandu can be modulated, with pressure applied by the heel of the foot. Other instruments include Katta sticks and clappers (used on the body of the drum); scrapers (corrugated sticks); shakas made from gourds (calabash); condensed milk tins and indeed any other instrument that can be fashioned from the environment. Hand-clapping weaves in and out contrapuntally with the singing and drumming.

Whylie suggests that, strange as it may seem, the music and dance of Africa has remained relatively pure in cases like Kumina, Gerreh and Ettu (other African core types), because many of the African traditions and customs were discouraged and, in some cases, banned. The Kumina practitioners, rather than relinquishing their inheritance, went underground. The drum rhythms and dance motions remained, therefore, intrinsically the same as when they had been brought from Africa.

The Kumina ritual is a core type of African retentions and as such serves the dual purposes of (i) providing clues as to the lives and the religious and social practices of our African ancestors; and (ii) reaffirming the complexity and highly developed state of the African religious and cultural practices – necessary for them to have survived in such a pure form through colonisation, creolisation and in many ways mere toleration by its own descendants, Jamaicans today.

The Kumina Technique

FIGURE 1

Position

a) The FEET are flat in first position parallel.
b) The KNEES are bent slightly.
c) The PELVIS is pushed forward.
d) The TORSO is arched back in line with the pelvis.
e) The HEAD is arched back or held upright.
f) The ARMS are pulled back behind the body. The elbows are bent allowing the forearms to come forward, hands palm upward beside hips. Henceforth referred to as 'argumentative position'.

Motion

Figures 1,2 & 4

a) The FEET are placed flat to the floor and retain contact with it throughout. The dancer moves forward by clenching his toes tightly together, creating a scoop or curve in the foot so that the heel and instep can move forward. When the heel is forward, the toes open wide to clench again over new ground. This motion of the feet, known as 'INCHING', is in itself very small. It is repeated a good number of times before much progress is made.
b) The KNEES are bent for better support of the body-weight as the dancer moves. They remain bent throughout.
c) The PELVIS is pushed forward and moves laterally from side to side on each beat of the 2/4 rhythm as the dancer progresses. The movement of the pelvis is sharp but relatively small in that the knees and feet do not separate to allow a wide dimension of swing. The dancer may accent one hip by giving more push.
d) Like the pelvis, the TORSO moves laterally from side to side on each beat of the 2/4 rhythm. The motion starts in the ribcage and this affects the shoulders and arms. (They do not move of their own accord except

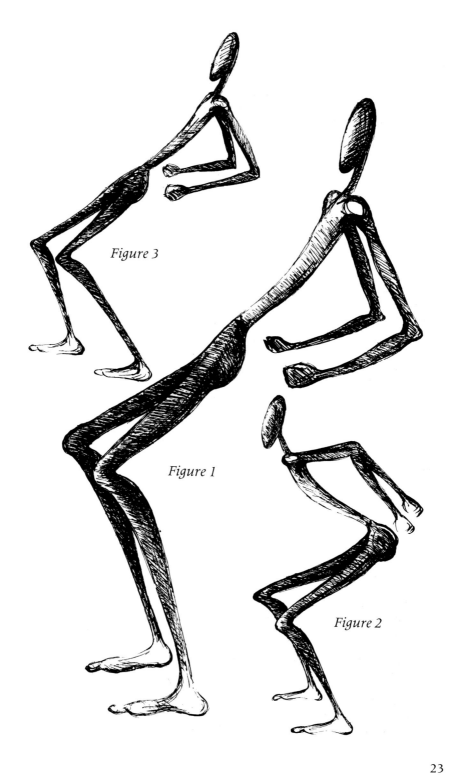

Figure 3

Figure 1

Figure 2

23

in Figure 4 where greater emphasis is placed on the shoulders being lifted and dropped alternately. The movement of the torso is accentuated by lifting one shoulder and inclining the head over to one side, away from the lifted shoulder. This is then repeated on the other side.)

e) The HEAD can be held in one still position or may give a slight shake from side to side like the torso.

f) ARMS retain their position in a relaxed manner.

FIGURE 2

Position

a & b) As for Figure 1.
c) The PELVIS is pushed back.
d) The TORSO is tilted forward in line with the pelvis.
e) The HEAD breaks the line created by pelvis and torso by tilting up to look straight ahead.
f) The ARMS are in 'argumentative position' (Figure 1).

Motion

See Figure 1

FIGURE 3

Position

a) The FEET are placed in a comfortable turned-out position on the floor with one foot forward of the other. The weight is placed on the back foot.

b–f) As for Figure 1.

Motion

a) The basic Kumina motion of the FEET is the same as for Figures 1 and 2. One major difference, however, is that the body-weight is placed not evenly between the legs but on the *back* foot. This of course affects the whole body stance – the back foot turns out slightly to help bear the weight and the back knee bends deeper than the front one. The feet still inch along, but the back foot pushes forward with greater emphasis, thus accentuating the change of weight.

b) The KNEES remain bent throughout.

c) The PELVIS still moves laterally but the weight on the back leg also allows it to move forward and backwards. While the accent is placed on the forward motion there is a heavy drop in the pelvis motion to the back.

d–f) As for Figures 1, 2 & 4.

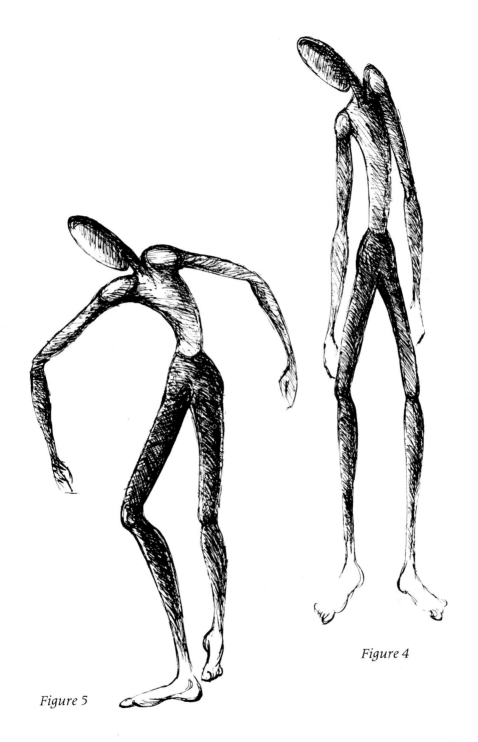

Figure 5

Figure 4

FIGURE 4

Position

a) The FEET are placed in a comfortable first position, heels slightly apart.
b) The KNEES are slightly bent.
c) The PELVIS is pushed slightly forward.
d) The TORSO is held in a slight arch back and tilted to one side (e.g. RIGHT).
e) The HEAD is tilted to the same side (e.g. RIGHT).
f) The ARMS hang beside the body.
g) The remaining (e.g. LEFT) SHOULDER is lifted, accentuating the tilt of the torso and head.

Motion

See Figure 1.

FIGURE 5: PIVOT TURN

Position

a) One FOOT is placed flat on the floor while the other is placed on the ball of the foot slightly behind.
b) The KNEES are bent.
c) The PELVIS is pushed back.
d) The TORSO is tilted forward in line with the pelvis.
e) The HEAD is either held down in line with the torso or is arched back to break the line of the body.
f) The ARMS are curved slightly and held out to the side, or pushed slightly behind the body.

Motion

a) The FOOT that is flat on the floor acts as a pivot. The heel is lifted continually and placed further forward to enable the dancer to move round. The other foot, placed on the ball, follows the pivoting foot round so that when the heel of the pivoting foot moves, the other foot is lifted and placed further forward or round also. This continual motion will form a turn.
b) The KNEES remain bent throughout.
c) The PELVIS moves laterally with an accent on one side.
d & e) As for Figures 1, 2 & 4.
f) The ARMS are basically held out to the side but the position is not rigid and the dancer is free to lower or raise his arms.

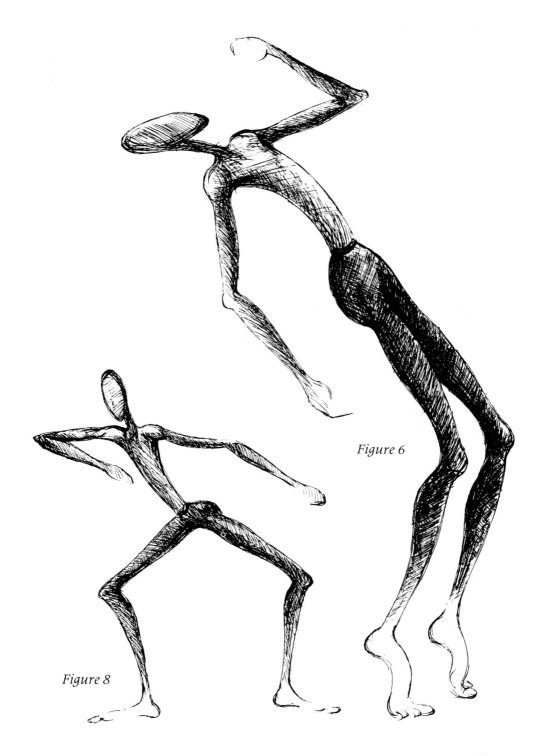

Figure 6

Figure 8

27

FIGURE 6: 'THE BREAK' – A Bamboche Step

Position

a) The FEET are placed flat on the floor *or* with the majority of the weight on the toes so that the heel is slightly lifted. The feet are parallel in second position.
b) The KNEES are bent.
c) The PELVIS is pushed far forward.
d) The TORSO is arched back.
e) The HEAD is held back.
f) One ARM is placed across the body at chest level. The other arm is curved and held out to the side slightly behind the body.

Motion

a & b) From being flat on the floor the dancer pushes all the body-weight way forward into the KNEES and onto the balls of the FEET. The heels lift off the floor.
c) The PELVIS is thrust as far forward as possible in one sharp movement.
d) The TORSO is thrown back as the pelvis pushes forward.
e) The HEAD is also thrown back.
f) The ARMS swing sharply across the body in one quick movement. The impulse is abruptly stopped at the same time as the body-weight is pushed forward – emphasising the sharp, quick quality of the movement. This 'break' occurs as just that: a 'break' to the continual motion of the pivot turn, for example, hence the sharpness of the motion. This taut position is held momentarily before resuming the previous motion.

FIGURE 7: 'THE ROLL TURN'

Position

a) The FEET are placed in a wide second position, turned out.
b) The KNEES are bent outwards, deep.
c) The PELVIS is pushed back and is almost on a line with the knees.
d) The TORSO is tilted forward.
e) The HEAD looks out to one side.
f) Both ELBOWS are bent and lifted up towards the sides of the head.

Motion

a) The FEET remain in a wide turned-out second position throughout. In order to complete the turn, the dancer jumps from one foot to the other, completing half-turns with each step.
b) The KNEES remain bent throughout so that the dancer travels on one level.
c & d) The PELVIS remains tilted back and the torso pitched forward throughout.
e) The HEAD keeps focus on a certain point towards which the dancer

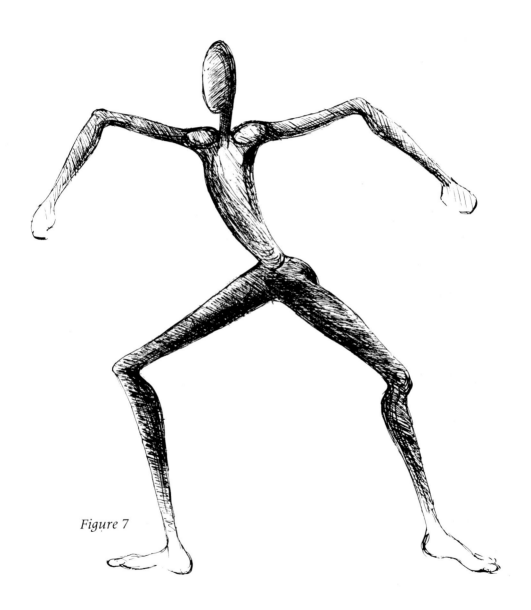

Figure 7

travels. Thus it will look over right then left shoulder alternately as the half-turns are completed.

f) The major focus of the Roll Turn lies in the ARMS. The bent elbows are pumped up and down as the dancer moves. The elbows are up when one foot touches the floor; mid-jump they are pushed down; then pushed up again as the other foot touches the floor.

FIGURE 8: THE WARRICK

Position

a) The FEET are placed in a wide turned-out second position.
b) The KNEES are bent, the majority of the weight being placed over one foot (e.g. RIGHT).
c) The PELVIS is tilted slightly back.
d) The TORSO is tilted forward and over towards the one side (e.g. RIGHT).
e) The HEAD looks out to the same side (e.g. RIGHT).
f) The leading (e.g. RIGHT) ELBOW is lifted out to the side and bent to allow the forearm to come back towards the chest. The point of the elbow is sharp and the arm angular. The left arm is held out to the side at torso level.

Motion

a) From a wide second position the dancer hops sideways onto the leading (e.g. RIGHT) FOOT. The hop is small and very low to the ground. (The majority of Kumina steps are earth-bound.) As the leading foot hops, the other foot brushes out to the side. The movement travels laterally. The feet keep their relationship to each other so that as one foot hops and the other brushes, the body travels slightly to the side. This is repeated rapidly and continually. The weight is mainly on the hopping foot.
b) The KNEES remain bent throughout so that the dancer travels on one level.
c & d) The PELVIS remains tilted back and the torso pitched forward and slightly over to the leading side throughout.
e) The HEAD looks over the leading shoulder throughout.
f) The leading ARM, with the elbow bent, is lifted up and down in sharp jutting movements. While the elbow is lifted the wrist pumps down. The motion is quick and the accent is on the upward motion. The other arm remains extended out to the side throughout. (The 'Warrick' is an adaptation of the fencer's position and motion while advancing.)

Variations on Basic Positions and Motions in Kumina

The Kumina is danced in a circle with dancers moving round in an anticlockwise direction. The individual dancers need not simply proceed forward but may move backwards for a while, shift slightly to the side to perform movements or 'break', i.e. perform a quick sharp movement contrary to what was being done before, at any time.

a) The basic Kumina position (Figures 1,2,3 & 4) is with both feet flat on the ground. The dancer 'inches' forward with the toes. Today's Kumina dancers, however – i.e. the younger generation – are sometimes seen to lift the heel of one foot off the floor so that while the flat foot continues to inch along, the lifted foot is used to *push* the body forward, thus facilitating easier and speedier progression. In Figure 3, for example, the *back* foot would be placed on the ball.

c & d) The basic Kumina motion (Figures 1,2,3,4, & 5) calls for a lateral shift of the torso and pelvis. (The pelvis may also move forward and backward for Figure 4.) Watching the older Kumina dancers it would seem that the torso and pelvic motions are small and subtle though very evident. Younger Kumina dancers, however, have developed the lateral shift into a rotatory pelvic and torso motion, completing wide circles with the torso and pelvis moving in opposition – i.e. both torso and pelvis perform circles in the same direction to the left or right but the torso goes against the pelvis so that when the pelvis is at the right side of the body, the torso is at the left and vice versa.

d) The arm position (argumentative) described in Figures 1,2 & 3 is commonly used for Kumina. However, the dancer is basically free to improvise arm movements at random. Other commonly used arms are: (a) The upper arms are held relatively close to the body while the lower arm is bent and held up so that the wrists face the shoulders. This position is most often used by the younger dancers while circling the torso and pelvis. This does give the Kumina a resemblance to the Dinkie Minie (below); (b) The arms may simply be carried at the sides of the body and react to the motion of the torso; (c) In Figure 6 any sharp movement of the arms may be used.

Dinkie Minie

Dinkie Minie is a member of the Wake Complex of traditional dances, mainly found in St Mary, St Ann and St Andrew, 3 parishes on the eastern side of the island. On the western side 'Gerreh', similar in content and context to Dinkie Minie, exists. The practice of keeping wakes is a tradition found both in Europe and Africa; the Scottish and Welsh settlers who came to Jamaica also practised this tradition. Wake ceremonies were, however, crucial to the African tradition:

> To the African tribesman, death and burial were perhaps the most important phase in a man's life cycle. On the funeral depended not only the prestige of those kin of the deceased surviving him, but the safe journey and status of the deceased in his new abode of the spirit world. It is not surprising, then, that the funeral rites of the West African slaves in Jamaica survived more than most other cultural elements.[6]

Thus, in some parishes, we can see where the master (Welsh or Scottish) and slave (African) shared customs.

With the African's particular situation in the Caribbean – uprooted from his homeland and forced into an alien environment and lifestyle – in an attempt at self preservation he held on even tighter to old customs. The African funerary rites were some of these. The Africans had always believed that in death one joined one's ancestors, and in Jamaica this belief was strengthened. They were convinced that the spirits of the dead returned to Africa and some slaves even took their own lives in an attempt to 'reach home'. In this foreign land, it became even more crucial that the dead person be properly and safely sent to join his ancestors – in Africa – where he could regain peace.

The African tradition involved the keeping of 'Set-Ups' and 'Ninth-Nights'. A Set-Up is quite literally that, a staying up throughout the night from the day of the death. Friends and colleagues of the bereaved will rally round the family to try and cheer their spirits. They will be encouraged to cry, so as to release their tensions, with songs such as:

> Bawl woman bawl, yu baby dead
> Bawl woman bawl, yu baby dead
> Bawl woman bawl,
> And ease your heart.

so that they will later be able to rejoice as the spirit is sent on its way.

The Set-Up lasts for eight nights and after the initial sadness it gradually becomes a rejoicing ceremony celebrating the fact that the deceased has moved into a better world. The first night of a Set-Up is the night of the actual death and the ceremony proceeds from there. The Set-Up is generally a boisterous event with much dancing and singing to lively mento music. On the third night of the Set-Up it is believed that the spirit of the deceased is raised from the body and may henceforth communicate with its descendants. Dinkie Minie, Ring Games (games in circular formation) and Role Playing become increasingly evident, finally climaxing on the eighth night. The ninth-night is the most significant, however, as it is then that the spirit of the deceased leaves the house to begin its journey 'home'. The Ninth-Night is a separate ritual within itself. The family of the deceased will 'turn-out' the spirit by turning over the mattress, rearranging the lay-out of the room and generally changing the habitual circumstances. The Ninth-Night is usually a more sombre occasion than a Set-Up, where particular regard is paid to tradition to ensure the spirit's journey is properly begun. Unlike the Set-Up songs, which are usually cheerful and topical, employing the Jamaican vernacular, old-time hymns such as 'Rock of Ages' are sung at Ninth-Nights. These are known as 'Sankeys'. Tracking, the practice of a leader reading the lines before the others sing, is common. Common also is the African practice of Antiphony – call and response. A major factor of the singing is that there is no rule to the way the harmony is employed; voices respond in unison sometimes and at others in harmony.[7]

The wake tradition therefore involves a week and more of activities. The whole community will often rally round for the Set-Up and Ninth-Night activities, taking on the responsibility of helping the bereaved family through this period, and encouraging them to rejoice in the journey of the spirit to the ancestral homeland. Part of the Ninth-Night activities includes feeding the dancers and singers, who will not hesitate to remind the householders of this duty. This is done in song:

> From me come ya me no see no founder [the owner of the
> dead yard or keeper of the Ninth-Night]
> From me come ya me no see no founder
> From me come ya me no see no founder
> Me a go mash up de booth and go wey
> Me a go mash up de booth and go wey
> Me a go mash up de booth and go wey
> Home a me yard.
> From me come ya me no get no caffee/white rum
> From me come ya me no get no caffee/white rum
> From me come ya me no get no caffee/white rum
> Me a go pull down de booth and go wey
> Me a go pull down de booth and go wey
> Me a go pull down de booth and go wey
>
> Home a me yard, yard, yard.[8]

Light refreshments are provided for the Set-Up, but a small feast is prepared for the Ninth-Night. This may consist of fried fish, coffee or chocolate, tea, crackers and bread. Some parishes will also serve curried goat and rice with Manish Water soup, made from the head of a goat. As the food is to be served, the singers may state their desires between the lines of a Sankey, e.g:

>   Rock of ages cleft for me
> (ASIDE: Two fish, two tea, two bread)
>   Let me hide myself in thee[9]

Meaning that they desire double helpings of food!

As with most folk forms, the instruments accompanying the songs are those which can be found. These include shakas, katta sticks, condensed milk tins, graters etc. The Tamboo, a cylindrical-shaped drum, is essential. Dinkie Minie is marked, however, by its use of an ancient string instrument: a fret-board made of bamboo and gourd and called a 'Benta'. The songs, both cheerful and sombre, play an important part.

The movement in Dinkie Minie focuses on the pelvic region, as Dinkie Minie is also performed in defiance of the death that has occurred. The dancers, male and female together, make suggestive rotations with the pelvis in an attempt to prove to 'death' that they are stronger than he, as they have the means with which to reproduce.

Cheryl Ryman writes:

> If we understand that procreation was/is considered vital to the African's survival in Life and Death, in Africa and the diaspora then we can perhaps understand their apparent pre-occupation with 'sexual movements'.[10]

Dinkie Minie and dances of the Wake Complex are singular in the West Indian tradition in that they were openly practised throughout the years of slavery and are still in evidence today. As such, they represent an unbroken line of tradition directly from Africa, Scotland and Wales to Jamaica today.

The Dinkie Minie Technique

FIGURE 9

Position

a) One FOOT is placed flat on the floor while the other is placed on the ball of the foot. (Note: just the *ball* beneath the big toe touches: the rest of the foot is so deeply flexed that both heel and all toes lift off.) The weight is on the flat foot.

b) The KNEES are 'knocked' together, i.e. the dancer closes his thighs together so that the knees meet. The lower leg is then separated as much as possible. As weight is placed on the flat foot the body leans to that side and the other foot is then furthest away from centre.

c) The PELVIS is pushed back and over to the side, to which the body leans.

d) The TORSO is tilted forward over the knees.

e) The HEAD breaks the line of the torso by looking straight ahead.

f) The ARMS are held in the 'argumentative' position: (Kumina Figure 1).

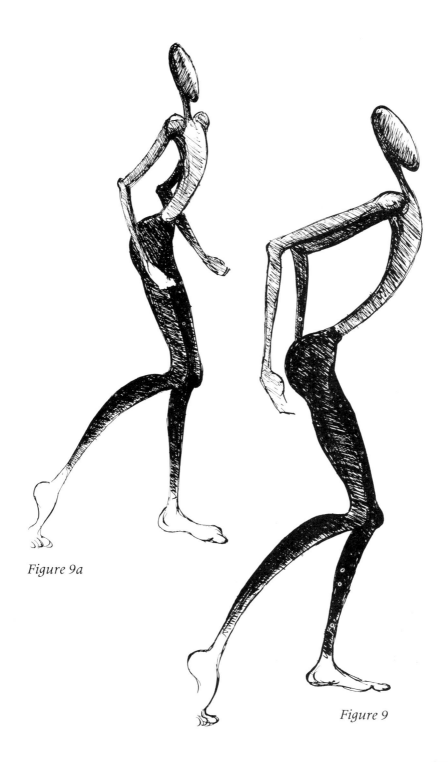

Figure 9a

Figure 9

Motion

Figures 9, 9a, 10, & 11

a)   The distinguishing characteristic of Dinkie Minie lies in the motion of the FEET. The working foot (i.e. the left), placed only on the very ball of the foot, brushes out sharply against the floor as the dancer moves. The movement is sharp and quick. The standing leg (i.e. the right), placed firmly on the whole foot, performs a low, quick, flat-footed hop, immediately before the working leg brushes off. Thus the standing foot gives the appearance of pushing the working foot onward.

b)   The KNEES keep as close together as possible as the dancer moves. Even while they may separate slightly as the working foot brushes off, the legs always turn in so that the knees face each other.

c & d)   The TORSO and pelvis perform rotatory motions as the dancer moves. They are circled once for each 'hop and brush-off' of the feet. Torso and PELVIS rotate in the same direction but touch opposite poles: when the torso is forward the pelvis is back; torso right, pelvis left etc.

e)   Dinkie Minie is a dance of defiance, thus it is common to see the dancer looking directly outward as if at the adversary – Death. However, particularly in Figure 11, where the dancer's arms are swung from side to side as he moves, the HEAD may reflect directional change.

f)   Figure 9: The ARMS remain in position behind the back and, without moving of their own volition, reflect the rotatory movement of the torso and shoulders.

Figure 9a shows a slight relaxation of the arms allowing the elbows to move forward.

Figure 10: The ARMS are held out to the side with forearms lifted, again reflecting the rotatory movement of the torso and shoulder. This results in the elbows executing small circles mid-air as the torso moves: forward, side, back, side.

Figure 11: These ARMS are used when the dancer travels to the side. Arms swing down in front of the body and up to one side for one pair of 'hop and brush-off' of the feet. The down motion of the arms is emphasised with a heaviness of limb. As the arms reach the other side, the elbows bend quickly to give a small break or flex to the motion before the arms are swung down again and over to the other side.

FIGURE 10

Position

a & b)   As for Figure 9.

c)   The PELVIS is pushed forward.

d)   The TORSO is tilted slightly back.

e)   The HEAD looks straight ahead.

f)   The ARMS are held up at the sides. Elbows bend to allow the forearms to lift up towards the shoulders. Palms face inward and fists are often used.

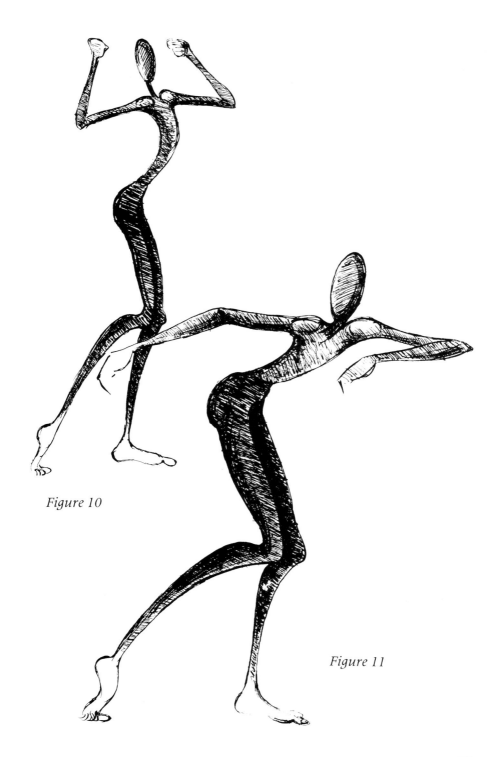

Figure 10

Figure 11

FIGURE 11

Position

a–d) As for Figure 9.
e) The HEAD can look straight ahead or over to one side.
f) The ARMS are held across the body to the same side. The elbows bend slightly so that the forearms lift up slightly.

FIGURE 12: 'BACKWARD PIVOT'

Position

a–c) As for Figure 9.
d) The TORSO is tilted back as much as the body will allow. It is also tilted as much as possible over to the side on which the weight is placed.
e) The HEAD is tilted over to the same side – the face may look straight ahead or down.
f) The ARMS hang loosely at the sides, elbows slightly pulled in towards the back. The shoulder of the standing leg is dropped lower than the other.

Motion

a) The FEET perform the basic 'hop and brush-off' of Dinkie Minie (Figure 9), but the standing leg is used as a pivot and hence hops on the spot as a circle or half-circle backward is completed with the working leg.
b) The KNEES remain close together throughout.
c) The PELVIS is pushed slightly backward with the left hip lifted.
d) The TORSO is tilted as far over the standing leg as possible.
e) The HEAD looks straight ahead or is tilted back.
f) The ARMS are moved by the motion of the torso. The 'break' to this backward pivot turn is a quick motion where the body hunches forward to counteract the backward movement. The arms are temporarily dropped and the head bowed before the dancer continues with the Dinkie Minie Backward Pivot.

FIGURE 13

Position

a) The standing FOOT is placed flat on the floor and takes the weight of the body. The working foot is placed slightly forward of the other. This foot is turned in and the ball of the foot only touches the floor (as in Figure 9).
b) The KNEES knock together as much as the forward foot (working leg) will allow.

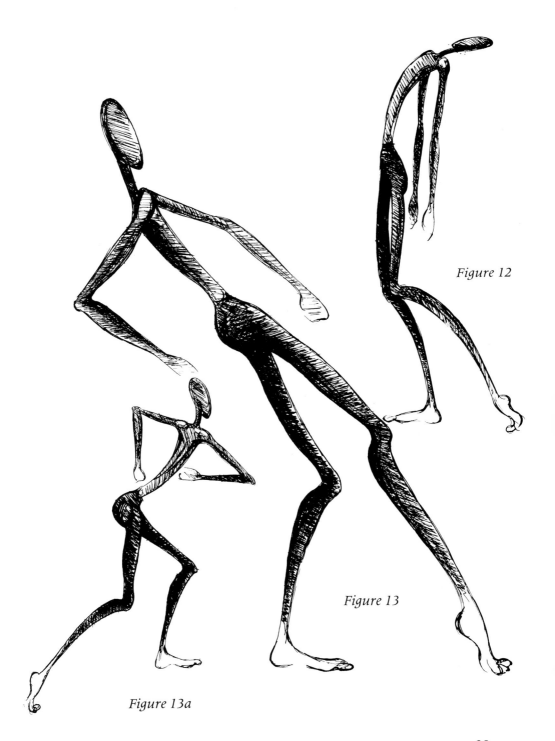

Figure 12

Figure 13

Figure 13a

c) The turned-in angle of the feet and knocked knees is carried into the PELVIS. The hip is pushed forward on a diagonal to the same side as the working leg. The outside of the thigh and hip are thus revealed.

d) The TORSO arches back on a slight angle to the same side as the working leg.

e) The HEAD looks straight forward.

f) The ARMS are held up at the sides. Elbows bend to allow the forearms to lift up towards the shoulders. Palms face down and fists are used.

g) The SHOULDERS are pulled up, causing the length of the torso to extend.

FIGURE 13a

Position

a) One FOOT is placed flat on the floor and takes the weight of the body. The other foot is placed slightly backward of the standing foot. Again, only the ball of the foot touches the floor (Figure 9).

b) The KNEES knock together as much as the backward foot will allow.

c) The PELVIS is tilted back and the hip of the working leg is pushed out to the side.

d) The TORSO is pitched forward of the pelvis.

e) The HEAD breaks the line by looking straight ahead or down.

f & g) As for Figure 13.

Motion

Figures 13 & 13a

a) This involves brushing the working leg forward and backward of the body alternately. The standing leg hops as usual so the only change is in the *placement* of the FEET in front and behind.

b) The KNEES stay close together throughout.

c) Rather than circling, the PELVIS is pushed forward as the working leg goes forward and bends back as the leg goes behind. The legs remain turned in so that the push forward of the hip is more prominent to the side of the working leg.

d) The TORSO, like the pelvis, tilts forward and back alternately: backward as the pelvis is pushed forward, and forward as the pelvis is pushed back.

e) The HEAD looks straight ahead.

f & g) The ARMS move from side to side at chest level across the body. As the left working leg is forward the arms are across the body to the same side and reverse when the leg is back. Rather than a smooth pathway the shoulders perform a slight lift and drop motion at each point of contact of the working leg with the floor. The arms reflect this slight hiccup in the shoulder.

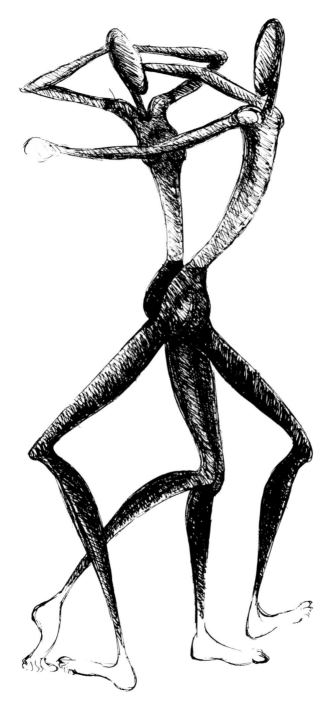

Figure 14

FIGURE 14

Position

This involves two dancers, one male, one female. They face each other and are very close.

a) The woman stands with her weight on one FOOT. The other FOOT is raised onto the ball.

b) The woman's KNEES are bent forward.
The man's knees are bent outwards astride the woman.

c) Both man and woman push their PELVIS forward towards each other – contact is very close.

d) Both man and woman lean back away from each other with the TORSO.

e) The HEADS look directly forward at each other.

f) The man's hands rest on the woman's shoulder and out to the side. The woman's hands are held behind her head.

Motion

a) Both sets of FEET remain on the ground.

b) The KNEES bend very low.

c) Both couples circle their PELVIS in one circle to the left or right side. Thus they move as one.

d) The TORSOS continue the circles individually.

e) The HEADS are held up to look at each other.

f) The ARMS, resting on shoulders and head, move as a reaction to the torso movement.

The Dinkie Minie, as part of the Wake Complex, is performed in defiance of death and this is revealed through the overtly sexual movements which are performed. Focus is confined to the pelvic area and when two dancers work together, the contact is very close. Two women may also dance together.

The knees remain bent and knocked together throughout (except for some coupling positions) and the working foot remains on the ball throughout. The style of the dance calls for bent knees and the body is usually twisted or bent. No straight line can be drawn from one body part to the other, as broken lines are used throughout. The body often leans away from the working leg when the dancer moves.

Variations on Basic Positions and Motions

Dinkie Minie is danced in celebration of a death and has no specific pathway. The dancers move about at will, meet with other dancers, separate and re-group. Much improvisation takes place, allowing dancers to express themselves personally through their movements.

a) When couples are dancing the man is sometimes seen to lift one leg up off the floor while still circling the pelvis and torso. Like all the coupling positions, this is overtly sexual.

b) Little variation occurs in the knees except in partner work where the knees may separate.

e) For each position or motion the dancer may use his head as he sees fit. Most often, however, the dancers look directly out – into the eyes of 'death'.

f) Improvisation is also allowed in the arms. A number of positions may be mixed at will (Figure 9a), or simply hang free. Dancers are sometimes seen with hands held behind the head, elbows out to the side.

1. Nettleford, 'Kumina', Jamaica School of Dance, May 1984.

2. *Ibid.*

3. Moncrieffe, Barry, Traditional Folk Forms, Jamaica School of Dance, October 1983.

4. *Jamaica Journal*, Volume 10, No. 1, p. 6.

5. Whylie, M., 'Traditional Folk Music and Dance', Jamaica School of Dance, 1984.

6. Patterson (1973), p. 195.

7. Whylie, *op.cit.*

8. Patricia Laing and Melinda Minott, first year students of the Jamaica School of Dance, from St Mary and St Thomas respectively. Discussions on Wake Traditions, June 1984.

9. *Ibid.*

10. *Jamaica Journal*, No. 44, p. 4.

CHAPTER TWO

European-Derived Dance Forms

Social: The Quadrille

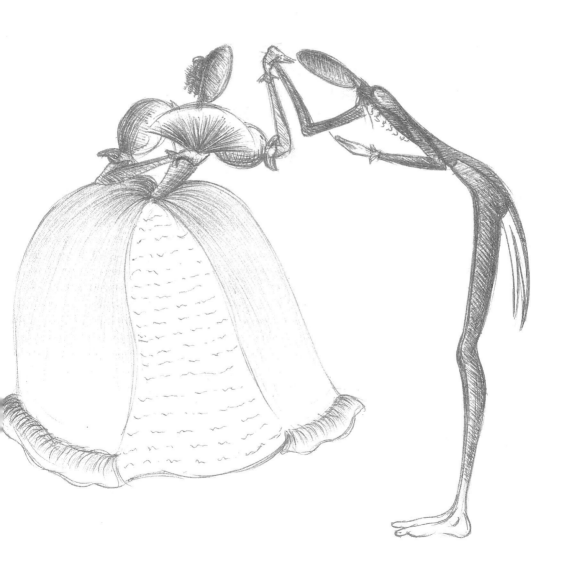

The Quadrille[1]

The precise origins of the Quadrille, an eighteenth-century popular dance, are somewhat vague, as writings of the time are not clear. Historians argue as to whether it originated in France or England. Curt Sachs (*World History of the Dance*) and Ivy Baxter (*Arts of an Island*), however, argue that, as France was the leading exponent of dance styles from the sixteenth century, it would naturally have originated there. The dance would then have been brought home to England by the Dancing Masters who frequently crossed the Channel from England to Europe in search of new dance styles. Other historians, however, would remind us that the French were not always the creators of the dance styles as they too sent their Dancing Masters to search out innovations from other countries. Regardless of origin, however, the Quadrille, like many of the other dances, was greatly refined and stylised in France.

Two general styles of dance existed at this time: dances of the court society and dances of the peasant society. While the peasant dances of the time emphasised fun and gaiety, using group work formations to emphasise solidarity and togetherness, the dances of the court, often stolen from the peasant forms, emphasised etiquette, manners and formality. The great flamboyance and the element of individual improvisation that the peasant forms allowed was disregarded here, giving preference to meticulous hand and head gestures, precise floor patterns and processional movements of the court. The dance was created more for effect and the appreciation of the onlooker than for the enjoyment of the participant. The Quadrille, as with all the court dances, involved a precise series of movements. Everyone learned the same steps from their dance tutors and performed them at balls, soirées and other appropriate occasions. All the dances of the time crossed the Channel with the Dancing Masters. Each country favoured its particular version of Quadrille, and thus a bounty of styles was evident.

Five basic elements were considered in the formation of a court dance such as the Quadrille:

1. Choral Dances Three types of choral dances (i.e. using movements in unison) were popular: the Longways Set, dancers placed in a column formation; the Round Set, formation of a circle or circles; the Square Set, formation of a square.

The emphasis within the choral dances was on group activity in unison. Recognisable figures such as the Square, Round and Longways were used as a means of displaying the group. The creativity lay not so much in body movement but rather in the different ways of moving from one formation to another.

2. Court Gestures Many gestures found in the Quadrille had come from the royal court society where much emphasis was given to highly sophisticated behaviour and meticulous etiquette. This resulted in numerous superfluous gestures of the body and limbs. Hands played an important part and were gloved for emphasis. The body was generally held erect and any bend thereof was stiff, particularly for the men, who maintained an almost military stance. The ladies were required to present or assume elegance. Thus, in the Quadrille, gentlemen held their left hands behind their backs while the right was held out for the ladies to place their hands. The lady either held out the skirt of her dress between thumb and forefinger or she held a fan. All gestures were stylised and meticulous.

3. *Partner Work* Various ways of working with two people were explored in composing the Quadrille. Partners could face each other; stand back to back; separate and return; walk forward and back together and endless other variations. Partner work was used to sub-divide the group and to help diversify the floor patterns. This would also allow for a little (subtle) flirtation between couples.

4. *Processions and Interweaving* The Quadrille incorporates dancers moving in a processional format from one place to another to change formation. The movement is gradual with as much emphasis given to the process of changing as to the actual end design. Formations like the 'Grand-Chain' and the 'Dosi-Do' require the dancers to interweave while changing places. The interweaving of dancers adds intricacy to the flow of the dance.

5. *Steps taken from the Peasant Dances of the Time* In the Quadrille, as with many court dances, certain steps are recognisably 'borrowed' from the peasant folk dances. The Dancing Masters would copy and then refine these steps, changing head and arm movements to give them the subtlety and grace required for a dance such as the Quadrille.

The Quadrille was brought to Jamaica in the eighteenth century when the Europeans began to settle there. Smith (1981) writes:

> In an effort to maintain a social status similar to that of the aristocrats in Britain, the white elite in the colony fashioned their lifestyle in keeping with their British counterparts. This was most evident in their manner of clothing (despite the hot climate); eating habits, housing, and above all, their manner of entertainment.[2]

The Quadrille was the most popular dance at the time in Europe and this naturally spilled over to the Caribbean. Its popularity was such that it was danced at all social occasions: weddings, balls and banquets held at the great houses on the islands. The slave population, particularly those house servants residing near the Great House, were able to watch and copy their master's dance. Funnily enough, because of its great emphasis on pomp and ceremony, which contrasted so severely with their own lives, the slave population learned and mastered the Quadrille also. An escape from the harshness of everyday life? Its popularity among the slave community grew just as it had in Europe. Though primarily adopted as a means of mimicking the master, the Quadrille was soon danced for its own sake at local gatherings, celebrations and on holidays such as Christmas, Easter and Crop-Over. Thus, in Jamaica, master and slave shared the same social dance.

In Europe, the Quadrille had taken on two distinctive styles, one very stately and refined, the other a livelier, more energetic version. This duality occurred in Jamaica also. The Jamaican 'Ballroom Style' Quadrille is based on the square formations of the European 'Cotillon', while the Jamaican 'Camp Style' Quadrille contains the Longways formation, variety and improvisation of 'La Contredance' from the European Quadrille. The Camp and Ballroom styles may use the same number of dancers but their performance styles differ greatly.

The Camp Style

1. The Camp Style is a bouncy Quadrille; the dancers are relaxed and enjoy themselves tremendously as they create and improvise with the movements of the dance.

2. The Camp Style is very earthbound in quality, reflecting the strong African influence of this style. The feet are placed flat to the floor. The 'bounce' quality, a very distinctive characteristic of Jamaican and, indeed, Caribbean dance, is retained and emphasised both in the knees and in the torso and arms, which bounce up and down as the steps are executed.

3. The dance has a spontaneous quality – improvisation is encouraged and participants are free to give individual style to their movements. This often gives a competitive element to the dance, as participants try to out-do each other. At these times, very intricate foot-work and stylised arm movements come into play. A mimicking of the European gestures.

4. The Camp Style was most popular in the rural areas of Jamaica where the country folk preferred its spontaneity.

The Ballroom Style

1. The Ballroom Style, a more rigid and set form, reveals a more refined quality and movement as the dancers glide from formation to formation.

2. The Ballroom Style retains the upward mobility of the Europeans. The body is held almost militarily formal.

3. Unity is stressed within the Ballroom Style. As emphasis is placed on the patterns being created, the group must move together for full effect.

4. The Ballroom Style was most popular in Kingston. Sophisticated Kingstonians could do a much better job of imitating the Europeans than could the rustic country folk who preferred to let their hair down.

5. The style reveals certain basic elements of the Caribbean folk technique – the torso is tilted forward with pelvis pushed back, or the pelvis pushed forward and the torso arched back. Pronounced use of the pelvis is made, particularly in the Mento figure where the pelvic movement is the centre of focus:

> Jamaican bodies, supple and responsive to rhythm, have carried the dance to the logical conclusion of hip-swinging syncopation.[3]

Also 'BREAKS', a temporary relaxation or cessation of the main movement, are common in the Camp Style. This comes originally from Africa.

5. The torso and pelvis are given only enough movement as would enhance the stately nature of the dance. The feet point whenever possible.

6. The costume for the Camp Style Quadrille is rustic. Head-ties and floral skirts for the women and colourful shirts for the men.

6. Costumes for the Ballroom Style are very formal. The ladies dress elegantly in long gowns, while men wear suits.

7. The music for the Camp Style, a basic 2/4, is played very fast, encouraging a freer dance style. As with most African music there are very few rests in the bar – the African style does not appreciate silence. In the Camp Style the African performance norm is used – the dancer never stands still but retains the bounce quality even while dancing on the spot. Syncopation is used to fill the gaps:

> Go in and out the window
> [syncopate:] *In Again*
> In and out the window[4]

7. The Ballroom Style Quadrille is danced to a basic 4/4 beat.

As with most Jamaican dances, instruments used were those that could be found or made. It was common, however, to have a guitar, fiddle and rhumba box. The main instrument was the fiddle, generally a hand-crafted, home-made version. Sometimes the piccolo, fife, saxophone or trombone

49

would lead the dance. Other instruments included the banjo, guitar, drum, marimba, double bass, and percussion instruments such as triangles, pieces of iron, forks, graters etc.

Most Jamaican folk dances reveal some evidence of pure West African, pure European and creolised elements. What vary are the particular quantities of these elements in each dance. The Quadrille retains the most European characteristics of all the Jamaican folk dances. In the Ballroom Style in particular, the European stance and style is rigidly imitated. The Camp Style, while showing greater evidence of some African characteristics, is still predominantly European in nature. All over Europe, even today, though no longer a popular social dance, the Quadrille is still being taught in dance schools and dance societies. In Jamaica also the Quadrille is no longer a social dance across the country. At the time of independence in 1962, the Quadrille was so popular that it was chosen as the national traditional dance of the country but, as with all the traditional dances, the Quadrille is seen less and less as a social dance and is now more of a historical dance form.

The Quadrille Figures

Unlike the other folk dances where a basic step or steps are indicative of the dance, each version of the Quadrille is a set dance from beginning to end. Each section is termed a 'FIGURE' and it is the dancer's role to learn and execute the FIGURES correctly. The examples of the Camp Style (below) are from the Parish of Portland.[5] The examples of the Ballroom Style are from the Parish of St Catherine.[6] For clarification of terms see Glossary (page 54).

THE CAMP STYLE

Formation – Rectangular Set

Figure 1
1. All couples 'Pass-through' to the opposite side, then repeat to regain former position.
2. All ladies execute a 'Figure-of-Eight' while gentlemen make small circles around the advancing ladies.
3. All dancers face respective partners and 'Balance', followed by a wheel.
4. Couples execute a 'Half-Promenade' around each other – on reaching opposite side, couples make small half-circle at this end.
5. Couples repeat 'Pass-through' to regain former positions.
6. Couples repeat stage three followed by the 'Honouring' of partners.

Figure 2
1. One gentleman and one lady of opposite couples in each set advance to centre and retreat.
2. The same pairs repeat the advance, circle each other and return to their former positions.

3. Stages one and two are repeated by the same pairs.
4. All couples 'Balance' and wheel.
5. Stages one to three are repeated by the other pairs of opposites.
6. All couples 'Balance' and wheel, followed by the 'Honouring' of partners.

Figure 3

1. As in Figure 2, one pair of opposites in each set advance to centre and dance together ('Balance').
2. The gentleman then takes the lady's left hand with his left hand 'Allemande' to collect their respective partners and move towards the opposite position.
3. The first pair again advance to the centre 'Balance' – gentlemen turn the ladies on spot – pairs return to their respective partners.
4. All couples 'Balance' and wheel.
5. All couples execute a 'Pass-through' to regain their original position.
6. The entire sequence is repeated with the other pairs of opposites dancing stages one to three.
7. The 'Honouring' of partners follows.

Figure 4

1. All couples advance to centre – gentlemen wheel opposite ladies. Couples then retreat to original positions in the Set – gentlemen wheel their own ladies.
2. All ladies execute a 'Figure-of-Eight' while gentlemen make a circle around them as they approach.
3. All couples execute a 'Pass-through' (called 'Fours' in Port Antonio), which is repeated.
4. All couples wheel – alternate couples wheel and stop while the other couples continue to wheel travelling to them. Gentlemen of moving couples hand their ladies over to the stationary gentlemen – the couples with additional ladies advance on the single gentlemen who in turn retreat. This advance and retreat is reversed – ladies are then handed over to the formerly single gentlemen and the advancing and retreating is repeated. Couples wheel back to their original positions.
5. All couples advance to centre, 'Balance' with opposites and gentlemen wheel opposite ladies to their (gents) home (original position in the dance).
6. Gentlemen cross over followed by ladies executing a 'Figure-of-Eight' (men also make a circle around them as they approach).
7. All couples 'Balance' and wheel followed by a repeat of stages four to six.
8. All couples 'Balance' and wheel followed by the 'Honouring'.

Figure 5

1. All couples hold hands and swing arms towards centre three times – gentlemen turn ladies on spot.

2. Ladies execute a 'Figure-of-Eight' while gentlemen do the customary circle around them as they approach.
3. Couples 'Pass-through' twice.
4. The crossing is repeated with one couple holding hands while the others separate and move on the outside of them (called 'Centre-Cut' in Port Antonio) – this is repeated with the former outside couples moving on the inside.
5. Stages one to four are repeated.
6. Couples do 'Mento' dancing on the spot for a few bars with own partners.
7. The 'Honouring' of partners follows.

BALLROOM STYLE

Formation – Square Set

Figure 1
1. At the end of the first musical bar all gentlemen step to the side and bow as the ladies curtsey. Couples 'Pass-through' and 'Promenade' around each other. On reaching the opposite side, couples make a small circle. They then repeat the 'Pass-through' to regain their former position.
2. Working couples execute a 'Pass-through', which is repeated by the same couples to regain their original position.
3. Working couples 'Balance' and wheel.
4. Ladies of working couples execute a 'Figure-of-Eight' around gentlemen, who make a circle around them as they approach.
5. Using the 'two-hand hold' the working couples execute a 'Half-Promenade' around each other – on reaching the opposite side, couples make a small circle. They then repeat the 'Pass-through' to regain their former position.
6. Working couples 'Balance' and wheel.
7. Couples 2 and 4 take over as the working couples and repeat the entire sequence.

Figure 2
1. The lady of couple 1 and the gentleman of couple 3 advance towards each other, then retreat.
2. The same pair cross each other to the opposite side (lady turns while moving).
3. Stages one and three are repeated by the same pair.
4. Couples 1 and 3 (working couples) 'Balance' and wheel.
5. Stages one to four are repeated with the other lady (couple 3) and gentleman (couple 1) of the working couples.
6. Couples 2 and 4 repeat the entire sequence as the working couples.

Figure 3

1. The lady of couple 1 and the gentleman of couple 3 advance towards each other, then retreat.
2. The same pair repeat their advance, hold each other's left hand (above their heads), circle and give right hands to respective partners. Maintaining hold of respective partner's hands, couples 'Half-Promenade' to opposite positions (i.e. side opposite their original position).
3. Same active pair again advance and retreat – on returning the lady turns on the spot, following this with a low curtsey, to which the gentleman responds with a bow.
4. Working couples advance to each other using a 'two-hand hold' but separate as they execute a 'Pass-through'. (Couples are now back in their original positions.)
5. Stages one to four are repeated with other lady and gentleman of the working couples.
6. As before, couples 2 and 4 repeat the entire sequence.

Figure 4

1. Ladies of working couples execute a 'Figure-of-Eight'.
2. Working couples 1 and 3 'Balance' and wheel.
3. Couple 3 will wheel for one bar and stop while couple 1 will wheel down to them. Couple 1 gentleman hands his lady over to couple 3 gentleman – this group (gentleman holding ladies on either side under arm) then advances and retreats on single gentleman, who in turn retreats and advances. Ladies switch over and the process is repeated. All join hands and make a half-circle in centre. Gentlemen then wheel opposite ladies to the ladies' respective positions.
4. Men cross over to their former positions while ladies execute a 'Figure-of-Eight'. (Men also do the normal circle as the ladies approach them.)
5. Working couples 'Balance' and wheel.
6. Stages three to five are repeated with couple 3 wheeling up to couple 1.
7. Couples 2 and 4 then take over, repeating the entire sequence.

Figure 5

1. All gentlemen hold ladies' right hands above their heads and turn them on the spot in front of them.
2. All couples wheel on the spot.
3. Ladies of working couples 1 and 3 execute a 'Figure-of-Eight' as the men execute their normal circle on their approach.
4. Working couples 'Balance' and wheel.
5. Ladies of working couples again execute a 'Figure-of-Eight'.
6. Working couples 'Pass-through' to opposite side, with one couple holding hands and passing on the inside while the other couple separate and pass on the outside of them – this is repeated in the reverse.
7. All couples repeat stage one.
8. Couples 2 and 4 then repeat the entire sequence from stage three.

GLOSSARY OF TERMS

Partner: Your initial partner. He/she will begin the dance beside you.

Advance: Walk forward.

Retreat: Walk backwards to place.

Balance: Step to the side with the right foot. Bring the left foot to join the right. Step to the side with the left foot. Bring in right to join the left. Repeat.

Pass-through: Walk forward and cross to the other side of the square. The gentlemen remain on the left, allowing the two ladies to pass side by side in the centre.

Wheel: The gentleman holds the lady in a waltz position, right arm out. Left hand on the lady's waist. He turns the lady round clockwise, on the spot or travelling, with a pivot step.

Promenade: A basic walk forward, the gentleman parading the lady to the opposite side and back to their original places.

Half-Promenade: The gentleman parades the lady to the opposite side.

Figure-of-Eight: Ladies dance creating the pathway of the number 'eight' as they circle around the men at both ends. Men complete half-circles around the ladies as they pass.

Arch: Partners or corners link outstretched arms, creating an arch through which dancers may pass.

Star: All dancers lift right or left hands up to the centre and move round in a circular formation.

Grand Chain: Weave in and out of the other dancers in regular pattern. Link left hand with partner then right hand with the next dancer. This is similar to the Maypole weave. (The Grand Chain is circular while the Longways Chain – Hey – uses lines.)

Dosi-Do: Walk forward toward opposite person, circle around opposite keeping backs facing, walk backwards to original place.

Honour: Gentlemen bow to ladies, who curtsey. This is usually done at the beginning and end of the dance or FIGURE. In the Ballroom Style, a slight inclination of the head may also be executed at the end of each figure.

1. Except where otherwise stated, this chapter is based on 'The Quadrille in Jamaica', a thesis by Andrea Smith (1981), Jamaica School of Dance.

2. Smith (1981), p. 15.

3. Baxter (1970), p. 201.

4. Whylie, M., 'Traditional Folk Music and Dance', Jamaica School of Dance, May 1984.

5. Source: Mrs Dorothy Bevan, dancer/trainer with Port Antonio Adult Cultural Group.

6. Source: Mrs Ivy Hin, dancer/trainer with Linstead Cultural Group.

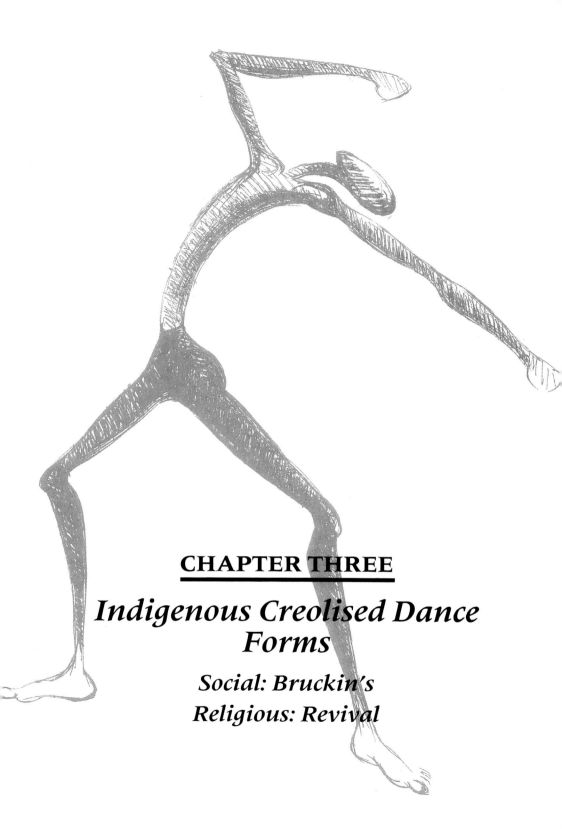

CHAPTER THREE

Indigenous Creolised Dance Forms

Social: Bruckin's
Religious: Revival

Bruckin's

B ruckin's is a member of the creolised group of traditional dances. As with Jonkonnu, the dance reveals a unique mixture of African and European influences. In Bruckin's, the pomp and ceremony of British royalty has been juxtaposed with African dance performance practices. The dance takes the form of a pageant – a bright processional parade of King, Queen, courtiers and other gentry. The movement, however, is mainly African-derived; the jutting forward of the pelvis, use of bent knees, flexed foot, tilted-back torso and bent arms are all elements attributable to the dances of West Africa. Bruckin's is unique in that this particular arrangement of African and British styles could only have evolved in Jamaica,[1] where its creators – the slaves – held in high regard their African ancestors, even while they learned to appreciate and indeed assimilate the favoured elements of British rule and British dance.

The original dance, 'Bruckin's Party', was a fully complex series of movements and sections. Beginning in August 1834, the dance was performed on 1 August each year in celebration of Emancipation. Bruckin's Party was a long processional dance, the participants moving gradually around the village in elaborate costumes representing the royal court. The dance made use of long, gliding steps with forward and backward movements of the body, movements said to have derived from the Pavanne, a European court dance of the fifteenth and sixteenth centuries. The Pavanne itself originated in Italy but was taken throughout Europe by the Dancing Masters of the time. The Pavanne was originally one of the more stately, processional court dances. Its slow, majestic pace made it suitable for the elaborate entrances of members into the court ballrooms. As such it was usually the first dance introducing the suite of court ballets for the evening. It was danced in 2/4 time and full court dress was worn (see Chapter Two: The Quadrille). This Pavanne would then have been brought to the Caribbean by Europeans, and passed on to the slaves in much the same way as the Quadrille. Also as with the Quadrille, the slaves 'creolised' the dance, making it more appropriate to their lives. The long, gliding steps and the pageantry of the dance were kept, as was the use of elaborate, stately costumes, but the upright stance of the Europeans was tilted far back on the diagonal: rather than keeping the torso stiff it was made to jerk in a purely African fashion, the foot was fully flexed and the subtle movement of the arms exaggerated to create a thrust.

Bruckin's Party would usually begin late in the evening. Dancers, formed in two sets, would proceed from one house to another, parading their costumes and displaying their dance skills. Each set, one in red, the other in blue, consisted of a King, Queen and courtiers, known as grand-sons and grand-daughters, sergeants, soldiers, pages etc. This was a direct imitation of what the newly-freed slaves saw as the Royal Family and the military complement that followed them. There was great rivalry between the two sets. Often the costumes, which were usually very elaborate designs imitative of court gowns, would be made in great secrecy and not revealed until the day of celebration. Props included crowns for the King and Queen and swords for the soldiers. The Queen of each set would first come out and dance for the duration of one song. This was a competition between the two Queens to see which could 'bruck' the better. Carolyn Smith writes:

> Bruck, as used in Jamaican creole, means 'to break' . . . [The dancer performs] a certain amount of movement in the lower region of the body which gives the appearance as if the body is broken at the waist.[2]

The competition would continue as the dancers proceeded around the village, the Kings and courtiers challenging each other as they went.

At around midnight, it would 'Tea-Time' and the song 'We are going out to the Supper Room' or something similar would be sung. Tea was held in a booth and gave the dancers a chance to rest. The European 'Tea-Meeting' tradition was a major part of the Tea-Break. 'Bidding' always took place. One member of the audience would be paid to perform a dance or song as entertainment. If the audience enjoyed the performance and wished to see more they would have to raise a bid for it. This could also work in reverse – if they wished the performer to leave the stage they would have to pay for this also. Bidding was an accepted method of fund-raising for the community. A second part of the Tea-Meeting ceremony was the section known as 'Show Bread'. This involved a kind of auction to provide a name for the ceremonial bread. Each name was accompanied by a bid and the highest bidder named the bread. A similar ceremony was held for the naming of the Queen. Throughout the ceremony speeches were made, introduced by the chairman of each set. These speeches, however, though rhythmically spoken, were full of any nonsense that came into their heads, without regard to coherence or thought, e.g.

> Ladies and Gentlemen,
> I am Parish Clarke and Section here,
> My name is Kaylem Totem,
> I am paid a blaze and auction sale,
> Big drum . . . I thank you all.[3]

The speech-making was also a competition, the winner being chosen by audience applause. In between speech-makers, and as an encore for the champion speech-maker, the swords would be run up and down the poles of the bamboo booths where the Tea-Meeting section was taking place. This was known as 'Razzling the sword'.

Today's 'Bruckin's' is a shorter version of Bruckin's Party. The pageantry of the original, with the King, Queen, courtiers etc. marching out to display their costumes and dancing skills remains, as do the long, gliding steps. The 'Tea-Meeting' section, however, with its tradition of bidding, speech-making and auctioning is uncommon now. The musical accompaniment for Bruckin's includes drums, knocking of the sticks, a fife and songs. The drummers and singers do not dance but move with the procession. The drums, rattling and bars, are played with sticks (showing a military influence) and worn hanging from the shoulders. The songs refer directly to the Emancipation of 1834, having been passed down from generation to generation. Songs include 'God Bless the Noble Queen Victoria Who Set The Nation Free', 'Recreation Around The Booth' and 'August Morning Come Again', which continues: 'This is the year of Jubilee, Queen Victoria set me free. This is the year of Jubilee'.[4]

Today, Bruckin's can only be found in one Jamaican parish, that of Portland. As with many of the Jamaican folk dances, particularly Bruckin's and the Quadrille, the culture is being kept alive largely through the Festival of the Arts, an annual celebration of Jamaican culture. Thus, from its original position as an integral part of Jamaican life and culture, Bruckin's – already a watered-down version of the original – is eroding still. At least exposure through the Jamaican Cultural Development Commission will allow its nature and content to be recorded before it dies out completely.

The Bruckin's Technique

FIGURE 15

Position

a)   The weight is firmly placed on one FOOT. The other foot is placed on the heel forward of the standing foot. The toes are flexed.
b)   The standing KNEE is bent, while the working leg is fully extended.
c)   The PELVIS is pushed forward.
d)   The TORSO is tilted back so that a diagonal line is created from the extended foot up to the head.
e)   The HEAD tilts back, keeping the line of the torso.
f)   The upper ARMS are held close to the torso. The elbows bend and the forearms are raised diagonally forward and up in front of the body. A fist is often used and palms face in toward the centre.

Motion

a & b)   From FEET placed together the dancer extends the working leg forward with the foot flexed so that only the heel touches the floor. As the working foot is extended, the standing KNEE bends to take the body- weight. Both legs are slightly turned out.
c)   As the working foot is extended, the PELVIS is thrust sharply forward and up. This motion can be small and suggestive or very large and overtly sexual.
d)   As the pelvis is pushed forward, the TORSO performs a 'bruck'. The back arches and then releases forward percussively. This appears like a jerk or shock in the torso region and, coupled with the pelvic thrust which occurs simultaneously, gives the whole body a snap movement.
e)   The chin lifts up and the HEAD lifts slightly as the release occurs.
f)   To emphasise the percussive motion of the body the upper ARMS are pulled sharply in to the side of the body while the forearms jerk slightly forward and out.

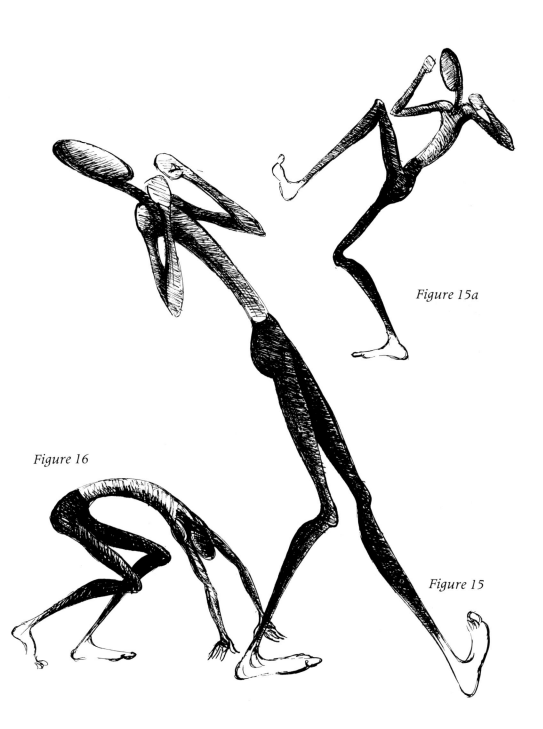

Figure 15a

Figure 16

Figure 15

61

FIGURE 15a

Motion (Variation)

Two styles exist: the 'decent march' (small movements of the pelvis as in Figure 15), and 'bruck back' (bigger movement of the pelvis and bigger movement generally). The dancer lifts the working leg quite high with a bent knee before taking a larger, lungeing step forward. This is then repeated on the other foot (Figure 15a).

FIGURE 16

Position

This position has a similarity to the crouched position of runners at the start of a race.

a) The working FOOT is placed behind the standing foot. The heel of the working foot is lifted so that the ball of the foot touches the floor. The majority of the weight is placed on the standing foot which is flat on the floor.

b) Both KNEES are bent.

c & d) The TORSO and PELVIS curve forward so that the upper body is hunched over the front leg. The whole body is close to the ground.

e) The HEAD curves over in line with the torso.

f) Both ARMS are curved and hang towards the floor. If the dancer goes very low, the hands may touch the floor.

Motion

a & b) From Figure 15 the extended leg is bent and pulled back towards the body. The FOOT, still flexed, passes the calf of the standing leg and is placed behind it on the ball of the foot as the working foot is lifted off the floor. To precipitate this movement there is a small hop on the standing leg.

c & d) The dancer contracts the whole body inwards, curving forward over the right leg as the left is passed back. While the standing arm is relaxed and curved at the side of the body, the left working arm, to complement the leg movement, performs a big sweeping movement down past the thighs and circles up behind the head to finish curved forward of the body. The hand may be placed on the floor. To return to Figure 15 the dancer may perform an outward turn on the front leg. The working foot is lifted off the floor with the knee bent. The arms lift upward mid-turn. The motion ends with the body in Figure 15. The working leg is extended. This upward movement of body and arms contains the upward mobility of the European influence in Bruckin's, which is a creolised core type.

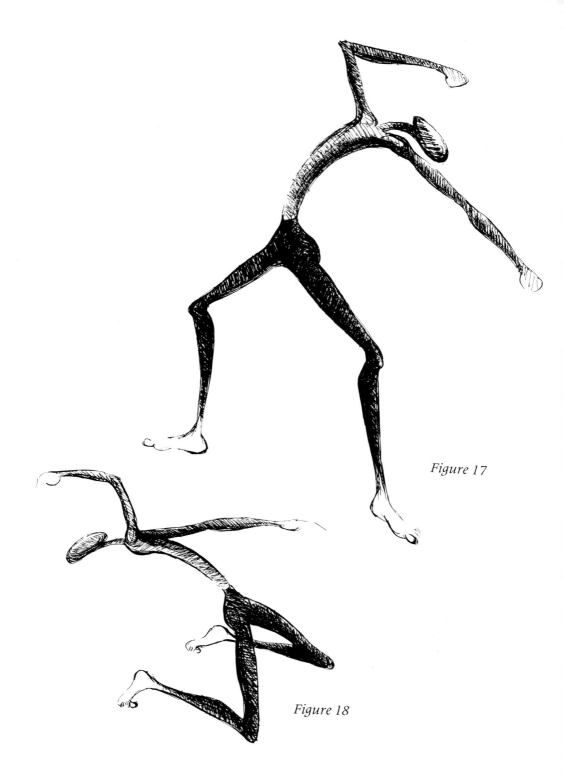

Figure 17

Figure 18

FIGURE 17: 'SILOH'

Position

a) Both FEET are firmly placed on the floor in a wide second position. The feet turn out.
b) Both KNEES bend as deeply as possible.
c) The PELVIS is thrust forward.
d) The TORSO is tilted as far back as possible. This can take the dancer way back so that the torso is almost parallel to the floor.
e) The HEAD is arched back in line with the torso.
f) The working ARM is held out to the side. The ELBOW is slightly bent to the broken line often evident in Jamaican/Caribbean folk dance. The other arm is curved and held in front of the body.

Motion

a & b) The FEET remain in a wide turned-out second position with the knees bent throughout. There is a slight flexion and release of the KNEES as the pelvis is thrust and released.
c) The dancer circles his PELVIS round in large circles, heavily accenting the forward position with a sharp thrust upward of the hips.
d) As with Figure 15, the upper body registers the shock of the pelvis thrust and the tilted back becomes taut.
e) The HEAD either looks directly out, thus breaking the line of the arched back, or it leans back in line with the spine.
f) One ARM completes a full circle up in front of the body, over the head and out to the side. The peak of the motion occurs when the arm reaches above the head and the pelvis is thrust forward at this point.

FIGURE 18

Position

a & b) The dancer kneels on the floor. Both KNEES are wide apart. The FEET are either stretched out behind or placed on the ball of the foot.
c) The thighs are lifted away from the calves as the PELVIS is pushed forward and upward.
d) The TORSO is arched back very low to the ground.
e) The HEAD arches back in line with the torso.
f) The ARMS are held as for Figure 17.

Motion

The dancer moves gradually from Figure 17 into Figure 18 and the basic elements of Figure 17 (the pelvic circle and thrust, the sweeping of the arm above the head) are retained. The difference occurs in the legs and feet. The dancer forces the body-weight lower and lower into the knees and diagonally downwards towards the floor. As he moves, the distance between thigh and calf is gradually shortened until the knees reach the floor. One knee is placed before the other so that the transition is smooth. The wide second position is retained so that the dancer ends on the floor with knees apart and legs extended behind him. The pelvis is lifted off the floor throughout, even while the back continues lowering itself to the floor in an arch.

Variations on basic positions and motions

Figure 15

The Bruckin's step can move the dancer forward or laterally. In the sideways step the body is turned towards the working leg on each step. The turn-out of the working leg is increased when the motion goes from side to side.

Figures 15 & 16

The dancer may perform two half-turns: after executing Figures 15 and 16 in succession (the working foot has been brought to the back), the dancer again picks up the working foot and executes a half-turn so that the body now faces the back and the working leg has been placed 'behind'. The dancer then picks up the standing leg and carries it in another outward half-turn round to the 'back'. The body now faces the front.

Figures 17 & 18

The arm movement for the Siloh is usually a big circling motion – 'lashing' – but sometimes the dancer uses a minimal circle, keeping the elbow bent and close to the body.

As a break from the pelvic thrust forward, the dancer sometimes stands on the spot, lightly bouncing up and down on one foot. The other leg, knee bent and forward, is lifted and the dancer 'gestures' with the foot. It is placed directly forward, to the side, across the body, out to the other side etc. Individuals use this as a chance to display style and finesse. This is known as the 'King Step'.

Revival

Revival is an Afro-Christian religion, originating in the late nineteenth century, the time of the Great Revival. In Jamaica today 'Revival' is actually one word used to reference two religious cults: Pocomania[5] and Zion. At first the term revival referred solely to the Zionist cult, which, of the two, bears more direct adherence to the doctrines of the Great Revival. Pocomania is now included in that term, however, as both cults evolved at the same time and from the same influences. Where they differed was in the precise amounts and the aspects of these influences assimilated. The Zionist cult is strong in Christian customs and practices, while Pocomania goes more deeply into African religious rites. Both, however, evolved as direct products of three major influences.

The first major influence on the evolution of Zion and Pocomania was that of the Baptist Movement. From around 1780, after the American Revolutionary period, Baptist missionaries such as George Lisle, George Lewis, George Gibbes and Moses Baker left the United States and came to Jamaica with the notion of coverting the African slaves to Christianity. Under their guidance, small Baptist churches were started in many communities, headed by local leaders (often black men as this was important for easy acceptance). The people took on a certain amount of the Baptist teaching, but soon adapted its dictums and practices to suit their particular needs and lifestyles. Laukenstein, in his article entitled 'Racial Values in Aframerican Music' writes:

> The negro insisted upon making a choice, that choice was determined by the demands of his perceptual consciousness for the exercise of which he found plenty of room in current Methodist and Baptist beliefs and practices. And as he chose those particular types of Christianity best suited to his needs, so he proceeded to choose the *elements* which were to make up for him his particular type of Methodist and Baptist Religon.[6]

Abstracting from alien themes to arrive at a more 'workable' version, suited to themselves, was something that the Caribbean slaves had been doing for years (creolisation) and their descendants continued to do. It was relatively simply for the slaves to adopt and adapt the Baptist beliefs as some were quite similar to the African creeds of their ancestors: firstly, dreams and visions as prerequisites for conversion to the faith were in keeping with the African belief that spirits could communicate with them. Also, the practice of submerging the body in water as a means of cleansing it of sin was also common to both Baptist and African ideology (the Baptist even believing that John the Baptist was more important than Jesus). Thirdly, the Baptists preached the notion of spirit possession, stating that the human body could be taken over by external forces. The Baptists also believed in the practice of anointing the sick for healing purposes. Both the notion of spirit possession and anointing of the sick bear close links with the African tradition of Myalism.

The second influence on Revival was 'The Great Revival'. It had begun in America in 1857 as a fanatical cross-country wave of religious fervour, spreading to Jamaica by 1860-61. Religion became the focal point of life, with people attending church services morning and evening, constantly showing repentance for their sins. The Zionist cult is directly linked with the early stages of the Great Revival in 1860 when the surge was still predominantly Christian-orientated. By 1861 in Jamaica, the Great Revival had assimilated many African modes and Pocomania is said to have been derived at this stage of the phenomenon.[7] Patterson writes:

> At first, the religious upheaval was glady received by the orthodox non-conformists (Baptists) and even by the Anglican clergy. But suddenly the whole movement 'turned African'. Myalism and native Baptism converged and in doing so shattered the hopes of the orthodox christians while laying the foundation for modern Jamaican revivalism.[8]

Myalism, the African religion that was brought into the Great Revival by 1861, was the third influence on Revival in Jamaica. Myal is distinctly African in content and context and one of the oldest artefacts of African religion, involving the powers of magic transmitted to the practitioner through spirit possession. As in Kumina (Chapter One), which is a by-product of Myal, possession occurs through a ritual of dancing and chanting and singing until the head is light, giving the spirit room to enter. When filled with the spirit, the Myal practitioner is said to have tremendous healing powers and can be applied to for help.

During slavery the practice of Myal had had to be performed in secret. After Emancipation in 1834, however, slaves were essentially free to choose their own paths in life and this included religious practices. Thus, the first direct and overt break from the orthodox Christian religion could be made: this was done through Myal ceremonies, and rituals were now openly performed. Years of Christianity and the very puritan notions of the Baptist religion had left their mark, however, and many people, rather than relinquishing either, combined the two. Thus Revival was born.

THE RITUAL OF REVIVAL

Edward Seaga in his study 'Revival Cults in Jamaica' (*Jamaica Journal*, Vol. 3, No. 2, June 1969) identifies three major ritual forms in Revival:

1. Prayer Meetings: Prayer Meetings are group gatherings mainly held for spiritual indoctrination, discussions of the functions and activities related to the group, for general worship of the supernatural powers or spirits, prayers, songs and/or Bible reading. Possession by the spirits at a Prayer Meeting is uncommon.

2. Street Meetings: Street Meetings are held to solicit new members and collect money for the group. On Saturday and Sunday nights in Kingston many Revival bands can be seen. Small groups congregate downtown or at Cross-Roads, Barbican Square, Half-Way Tree or Papine Market – wherever they will get an audience. The group can be distinguished from afar by the rhythmic dancing, drumming and preaching and singing, complemented by the interjections of Bible readings. Onlookers surround the groups and collections are taken up.

3. Rituals for Specific Purposes: May include 'Feasting Tables' 'Altars' and 'Baths'. 'Feasting Tables' (sometimes known as 'Duties') are held for specific instances within the community, from regular yearly celebrations to spontaneous events, such as healing, mourning and memorial services. The rituals are called 'Tables', as a table is laid containing mediums through which the desired spirits may travel. Like Kumina, the mediums may include rum, water, flowers, candles etc. The colour of the table-cloth and the exact mediums used will indicate the purpose of the ritual. (In Zion, an actual table is used, covered with a cloth. In Pocomania, however, it is more common to simply draw a circle on the earth, cover the ground with a cloth and place the mediums on top.) Both Pocomania and Zionist groups combine Bible reading, preaching, singing and movement in these rituals, invoking the spirits to enter the ceremony and fulfil the desired purpose.

In Puk-kumina, Feasting Tables begin on Sunday nights. A table with fruits, candles, drinks (alcoholic and carbonated), bread, vegetables, cooked food, and flowers is spread. The Sunday night is devoted primarily to speech-making by hosts and visitors on the purpose of the function, mingled with much singing and a little Bible reading and prayer. At roughly midnight the table is 'broken', that is, its contents are distributed among those present with some being set apart for the spirits after the candles are all lit. After this, there is usually some labouring (Trumping) until near dawn. For revivalists, the most important part of the programme begins on Monday evening when the 'bands' travels in the spirit world. This continues until about 3 am to 4 am on Tuesday. On Tuesday evening the sacrifice is held, and travelling is resumed Tuesday night until Wednesday, when the feast is held.[9]

Baxter (1970) writes that the pattern of the ritual (Pocomania, but this applies also to Zion) is that of singing interspersed with preaching and Bible reading, led by the Leader or Shepherd, until certain members 'get into the spirit'. Musical accompaniment for the singing consists of drums: a large bass drum, worn over the shoulder and beaten with one large padded stick (showing a military influence) and a kettle drum, hit with sticks. A tambourine, shakas and other basic percussion instruments will be played by individuals in the band. The basic rhythm of the bass drum is 4/4: 3 even beats and a rest. The kettle drum 'speaks' – i.e. it carries the melody.

Baxter identifies three steps towards possession:[10] Trumping,[11] Wheeling and Possession.

1. Trumping: Trumping is essential in the build-up to 'possession'. The Tumping section occurs after the singing and Bible reading and involves the members moving steadily round in an anticlockwise circle (Figure 19, below). The bodies bend forward as the members move and at the same time the forward step is accented with a heavy exhalation of the breath. In this exhalation, the air is forcibly pushed from the body so that a heavy guttural groan emanates. Each bend is accompanied by an exhalation groan, with the inhalation groan on the up-swing, setting a 2/4 beat. This beat sets the rhythm for the accompanying music. Seaga also stipulates that the Trumping step differs between the two groups:

> The bowing of the body to the accompaniment of groans is absent here [in Zion] in contrast with Pukkumina. Instead the motion is side-stepping. The body is raised a tip-toe on one foot and then vigorously, stampingly lowered on the other; at the same time the downward foot is usually moved sideways with a slight hop in that direction.[12]

The Trumping is lead by the 'Shepherd' in Pocomania and the 'Leader' in Zion. From the centre of the group he 'CYMBALS', i.e. he complements the beat of the Trumping by reciting 'in tongues' or nonsense syllables. These take the form of a chant. By the end of the Trumping stage the drums are often stopped so the only sounds heard are the guttural sounds and 'cymballing' of the Leader or Shepherd.

2. Wheeling: The Wheeling stage comes between Trumping and Possession. The body is held low and bent forward as the feet move rapidly round on the spot. The body equilibrium is maintained between spinning spells by statue-like poses, dynamic semi-falls towards the floor and snappy restorations of balance.

3. Possession: In Pocomania the onset of the possession state is usually experienced by paralytic shock in one leg followed by a recession of consciousness.[13] Members are possessed by the Earth-bound Spirits; when consciousness is regained, the possessed travels through the spirit world. A circle is formed as each imitates in movement and sound the particular spirit that has possessed him or her – e.g. if possessed by the Dove spirit, then dove movements and cooing sounds will emanate; if possessed by the Bell Ringer spirit then the Bell Ringer movement (Figure 23) will be seen.

In Zion, unlike Pocomania, members are possessed solely by Heavenly Spirits and Archangels. Possession can be marked by the harmonious groaning of the members, the sounds of which are said to further attract the spirits.

Zionists call possession 'receiving messages'. Only the Leaders or those who hold high positions in the groups are expected to understand the messages sent by the spirits. Therefore the Leader's role is often concentrated on interpreting the messages received. To facilitate this, he has first to organise the members who have 'caught the spirit', generally in a circle, and then drill them in the side-step and groaning pattern (see 'Trumping'). All groan on the particular beat he sets, then change to another and continue changing until he feels that all those encircling him are now possessed to the same degree as himself. At this point it is believed that all the group are in full harmony and therefore can communicate with each other through the spirit. The Leader reveals the message by singing short, improvised melodies in the 'unknown tóngue'. The melodies created make striking and beautiful use of polyrhythms. Rather than being translated into words, the message is said to be one of prosperity if the singing of the possessed is harmonious. If unharmonious the message is said to be evil.

In both cults possession is a limitless phenomenon, lasting anything from minutes to days. Throughout possession the body is completely taken over by the spirits and the person is totally unaware of his environment and his actions. Often a large number of members get possessed simultaneously and it is then the job of the Leader or Shepherd to maintain control. Others who are not possessed keep up the singing.

SOME SIMILARITIES WITHIN POCOMANIA AND ZION

- Both groups have roots in both African and Christian religious practices.
- Individual groups are referred to as 'Bands'
- Both sects are committed to their religion and can be said to 'live Revival', as from this source they obtain hope and faith to keep going when all else has failed.
- The place of worship is known as a Site and is marked by flags. Bright and colourful flags are flown to attract the spirits and to identify the place as a Revival ground. Zion sometimes uses buildings or old churches for its Site.
- The most sacred area of the Site is known as the Seal. In Pocomania this area is located outside, around a central pole, while in Zion it is usually in the mission house. The Sites are well screened. In Pocomania they are at the top of a hill. Meetings are held outside, usually on the ground so as to be as close, as possible to the earthly spirits.
- Some Sites are covered but the Seal is always bare.
- Articles found on the Site: benches; a table spread with a white or coloured cloth (depending on the occasion); flowers; Bibles; hymnals; candles; water and food. In Pocomania the yard will usually have a water pool or at least an earthenware jug filled with water. Like cream soda, water is important as a medium for calling the spirits. Huts, called Offices, are also evident, being used for consultation with clients seeking healing or advice.
- Before entering the Site, participants are required to 'turn a roll', i.e. turn round on the spot.
- During possession the alphabet sometimes comes into play. Letters can sometimes be distinguished as the dancers groan and stamp their feet. Numbers also come into play. These numbers and letters come to the participants through inspirational visions seen by them and used to quote Bible references, give prophetic revelations etc. The full meaning of the numbers and letters are interpreted through the ancestral or spiritual powers of the members in possession. Interpretations could be literal, e.g. 'B' for Bible and the number '6' to indicate the month of the year or 6th chapter in the Bible. Members relate the numbers and letters to the event for which the ceremony is taking place.
- Members of the hierarchy: in Zion the Leader is also known as the 'Captain', if male, and 'Mother' if female. Next in line is the 'Armour

Bearer', then 'Deacons' and 'Elders', who aid in the affairs of the bands, Baptism and Communion etc. Some 'Functionaries' take the name of a particular spirit and are given special powers to command and rid others of their particular name spirits – Dove Cutter, Hunter, Sawyer, Planner, Messenger, Bell-Ringer etc.
● Rituals: for healing or Obea. In Pocomania only, a prayer meeting or table is held. To combat any social problems, a street meeting will be held out in the community. This is also an opportunity to acquire new members.
● 'Baths' are sought by individuals with specific problems. They would be stripped and covered with a mixture of water, milk, coconut water and any other substances thought appropriate for each particular case. The substance is allowed to dry on the body for continued effect.
● Both Pocomania and Zion believe in the supernatural powers of the spirits. The Pantheon of spirits include: Heavenly Spirits – Divine God, Archangels, Angels, Saints, Bible Prophets and Apostles; Earth-Bound Spirits – Satanic Powers, Fallen Angels; Ground Spirits – The Human Dead (ancestors).
● Each spirit (except Divine God) has a preference in colour, food, drink, music, etc., and the Shepherds and members have to acknowledge these preferences in calling the spirits.
● The supernatural world is thought to be similar to the natural world, including countries with rivers, lakes, forests, mountains, etc. The spirits live as humans do, eating, drinking and attending church services.
● Individuals are believed to have a dual soul – one roams around while the other sleeps. After death one remains by the graveside while the other journeys to Heaven or Hell.

SOME DIFFERENCES WITHIN POCOMANIA AND ZION

Many differences between the two sects have already been pointed out in the previous pages, e.g. differences in level and type of influence, the nature of possession etc. The cults can further be separated:
● The Zion Pantheon of spirits gives hardly any recognition to the Earth-Bound and Ground spirits. While not denying their existence, Zionists view these spirits as evil, with negative powers. Instead they concentrate on the Heavenly and Biblical spirits – Archangels, Apostles and Prophets. This is indicative of the Baptist–Christian influence, stressing the Triad as the focus of worship. In Pocomania the Earth-Bound and Ground spirits are acknowledged and catered for. Certain spots on the site will contain mediums, e.g. water, crotons, cream-soda, etc., specifically to encourage the presence of these ancestral spirits, whom they firmly believe are working for them. (This shows the African-Ashanti influence.) The Heavenly Spirits are thought to be too busy to cater to their everyday needs.
● In Zion, while each band will have its Leader, there is no single Leader who presides over the entire cult. In Pocomania the Sitting Cronen Shepherd presides over the entire bands. As well as leading the singing and controlling the possession stage, his function is to crown the Post Holder and Leader of each bands.

• At the trumping stage, Zionists maintain a regular circle, moving anticlockwise. In Pocomania, a horse-shoe formation is maintained, members being careful to leave a space through which the spirits may enter.

• In Zion, sacrifices are virtually non-existent as the members deal with the Heavenly Spirits. In Pocomania, sacrifices are made every Tuesday. As part of the Libation process, a goat is killed and its head removed. The blood, along with white rum and cream-soda (strong mediums through which spirits travel) are used to appease the spirits.

COLOURS USED IN REVIVAL RITUALS

Green: healing; success; marriage.
Yellow: transformations; the colour is thought to be very holy and is used in intellectual cases.
Red: love; to ward off destruction.
White: purity; thanksgiving.
Blue: motherhood; symbolic of Mother Mary.
Gold: holy; source of power.
Black: for destruction; to kill or hurt.
Purple: order of sanctification; new membership.

Two major centres for Revivalism exist today, Blake's Pen in Mandeville, Manchester, and Watt Town in St Ann. Blake's Pen is mainly regarded as a *healing* centre and is visited by thousands each year; believers and non-believers alike seek the services of the 'healers'. These are people blessed with special power to heal or to look into the past or future. Mondays each week are particular days for healing. (Zionist are generally thought to be the better healers of the two cults.) Watt Town is the *spiritual* centre for Revival. It is the Mecca for Revivalists who journey there on the first Thursday in March each year for a convention-type gathering.

Today, Revivalism is, for most people, not simply a religion but a way of life. No clear distinction is made between church and life because the religion is functional and Revivalists practice what they preach. The religious beliefs have come to be the core of life around which everything must revolve: thus it is more important for a Revivalist to attend a 'Table' than to attend to other duties. This motion clashes with modern thinking, but what is to be done with a person who, being possessed, is not even conscious of her environment much less her duties within it? Revival is still to be found amongst the lower strata of society, particularly Pocomania with its African retentions. As such it is present but often ignored by the rest of Jamaican society. Even though many people from the upper strata of society are secret Revivalists, it is not openly welcomed. The colourful and boisterous marching bands seen in down-town Kingston, and the packed-full coaches in the rural areas, are tolerated but not encouraged; many feel that the sobriety of the Anglican religion is the only 'respectable' method of worship. It is patently obvious, however, that Revival offers a more tactile, more total method of emotional release than can be found in the average church. If it is to remain with the lower classes, the 'roots' people of Jamaica, then so be it, as they give full value and appreciation to their culture and welcome the emotional release Revival offers.

The Revival Technique

FIGURE 19: 'Trumping'/Drilling Step/Labouring

Position

a) The right foot is placed slightly in front of the left. Both FEET are parallel and flat to the floor.

b) While the left KNEE remains straight, the right knee bends forward with a slight turn in. The majority of the weight is over the right knee and foot.

c) The PELVIS is slightly back but curves naturally round to the right as the knee is bent.

d) The upper body is curved and leans over the working (right) leg. The TORSO turns slightly inwards towards the standing (left) leg, so that the dancer almost takes up a sideways position.

e) The HEAD follows the line of the torso by also turning in towards the standing leg.

f & g) The right SHOULDER is pushed forward, allowing the ARM to curve slightly; the palm faces back, while the left arm hangs freely by the side.

Motion

a) From the standing position with both FEET together, the dancer places the right foot forward, shifting the body-weight onto this foot. The left foot remains in place.

b) While the left KNEE remains straight, the right knee bends as the foot is moved forward.

c) The PELVIS shifts slightly to the right side as the foot lunges forward.

d) The TORSO curves over and round to the right side with the movement of the foot forward.

e) The HEAD turns towards the left shoulder.

f & g) The right SHOULDER is pushed forward, causing the ARM to curve slightly.

All movements are done simultaneously on one count.

FIGURE 19a

Position

a) Both FEET are placed firmly on the ground, parallel, in a natural standing position.
b) Both KNEES are straight.
c & d) The PELVIS and TORSO remain naturally erect.
e) The HEAD looks forward or over the right shoulder.
f) ARMS hang slightly behind the body.
g) While the left SHOULDER remains straight, the right shoulder is pulled back and down.

Motion

a) The left leg is brought forward to meet the right, which remains forward.
b) As the left FOOT joins the right, the KNEE straightens so that the body straightens up.
c) The PELVIS moves naturally as the left foot is brought forward.
d) As the left leg joins the right, the TORSO straightens out to face straight ahead.
e) The HEAD looks straight ahead.
f & g) The SHOULDER is pulled sharply back. The ARM relaxes and hangs slightly behind the line of the body.

All movements are done simultaneously on one count.

FIGURE 20

Position

a) Both FEET are turned-out and slightly apart. The dancer lifts the heels off the floor so that the weight is transferred to the front of the foot (relevé).
b) Both KNEES are straightened.
c) The PELVIS remains naturally erect.
d) The TORSO is lifted slightly, continuing the upward movement started in the feet.
e) The HEAD is tilted back and the face looks up to the skies.
f) Both ARMS are fully extended above the head creating a V-shape with palms forward and fingers spread.

Motion

a & b) From standing flat on both FEET, the dancer lifts the weight off the heels to rise forward onto the toes. The KNEES bend, better to facilitate this. The dancer may either rise sharply onto the toes or bend the knees deeply in preparation for a small jump into relevé.
c) The PELVIS retains its natural alignment, dropping back slightly as the knees bend, to straighten up as the dancer moves into relevé.

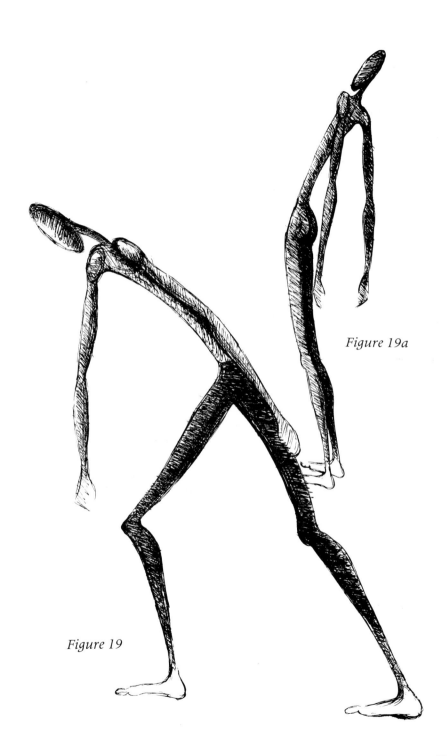

Figure 19a

Figure 19

75

d) The TORSO lifts up slightly as the dancer straightens the knees to begin the upward motion of the body.
e) The HEAD lifts up and arches back.
f) The ELBOWS bend slightly before straightening up above the head. The ARMS stretch in a V-shape, with fingers outspread.

The whole body is tense in its upwards stance. A slight shake of the body in this position often occurs.

FIGURE 20a

Position

a, b & c) As for Figure 20.
d) The TORSO, still lifted upward, is tilted over to the right or left side.
e) The HEAD follows the line of the torso, tilting over to the right or left side.
f) Both ARMS are fully extended up above the head. They too follow the tilt of the torso so that the V-shape is tilted over to the right or left side also. Palms are forward and fingers spread.

Motion

The motion is the same as for Figure 20 with the upper body tilting to either side.

FIGURE 21: 'WELCOME'

Position

a) The weight is placed over the left FOOT, which is flat to the floor.
b) Both KNEES are straightened.
c) The PELVIS remains in its natural relationship to knees and torso. It is neither forward nor back.
d) The TORSO is tilted over to the left side.
e) The HEAD keeps the line of the torso by inclining to the left also.
f) The ARMS hang at the side and do not move of their own volition but the tilting of the torso to the left naturally causes the arms to follow the line of that tilt.

Motion

Figures 21 & 21a
a) The dancer walks forward from one FOOT to the other. He emphasises the step onto the left foot by pausing for a fraction of a second before stepping onto the right.
b) The KNEES remain straight as the dancer moves, giving a certain rigidity to the motion.
c) The PELVIS moves naturally from side to side with the movement of the body.

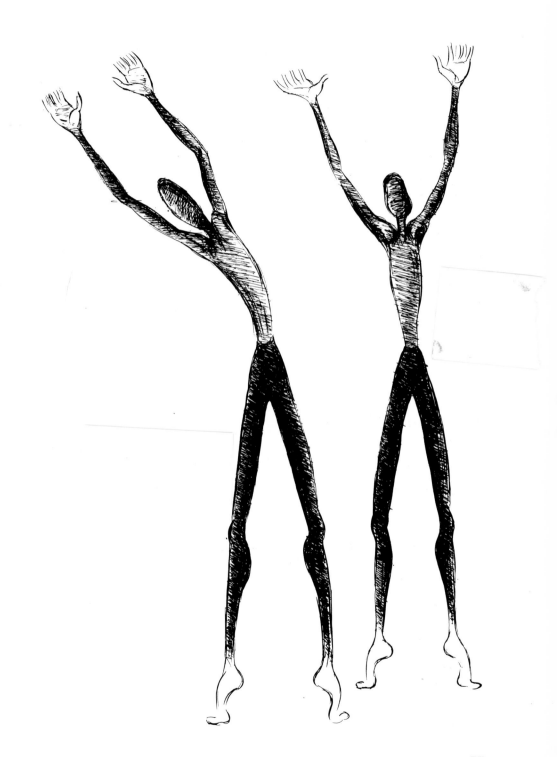

d)   As the left foot is placed forward, the TORSO is tilted over to the left side. The step on the right foot brings the torso back to the *centre* so that the motion is emphasised only to the left.
e)   The HEAD remains in line with the torso and thus tilts over to the left also.
f)   The HANDS remain in place by the side or with right hand lifted (a) and are affected by the tilt of the torso, causing them to shift over. With the right hand lifted, a slight tremor or shake of the hand may occur.

FIGURE 21a

Position

a, b, c, d & e)   As for Figure 21.
f)   The left ARM hangs naturally at the left side while the right arm is lifted out to the side with elbow bent so that the forearm is held up. The palm of the hand is forward and fingers are spread.

Motion
The motion is the same as for Figure 21.

POSSESSION

The dancer lies prostrate on the floor. Face upward or downward. The limbs are stretched and taut as the body vibrates. Arms are stretched in a 'V' above the head and fingers are spread. The head looks up or to either side. If the dancer lies face downwards, the head will be arched back to loop out or up.

Motion
Lying on the floor, the dancer shakes parts or the whole of the body from fingers to feet. It is a motion which indicates possession. The more possessed the dancer becomes the more energetic the vibrations. The dancer may 'break' by stopping still in a tense position. The dancer remains on the floor but may roll onto the side or back at will. This is a totally uncontrolled movement, intense and often wild. Usually, other participants are required to hold the possessed one down before the spirit is exorcised.

FIGURE 22

Position

a)   The dancer stands in a wide second position.
b)   The KNEES are bent.
c)   The PELVIS is pushed slightly back.
d)   The TORSO is pushed and *arched* as far forward as possible, giving an open look to the chest.
e)   The HEAD is thrown back so that the chin juts forward.

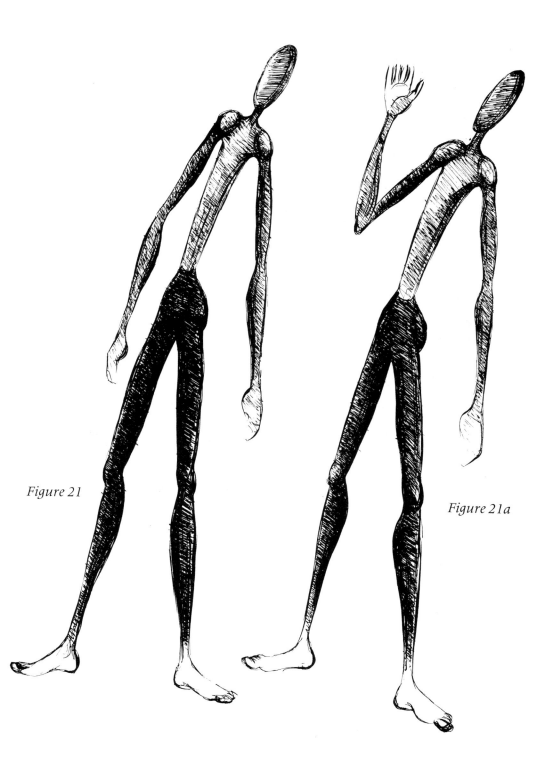

Figure 21

Figure 21a

f)   The upper ARMS are lifted, at chest level, to the side, away from the body. The ELBOWS are bent and pulled back beyond the arch of the torso. The lower arms are forward, palms face down.

Motion

a)   The dancer shifts the weight from one leg to the other while bouncing on the spot.
b)   As the weight is transferred, the KNEES bend deeper to take the weight of the body.
c)   The PELVIS is pushed back as the weight is transferred.
d)   The TORSO is arched to give an open chest and is pushed as far forward as possible in one quick movement as the weight is transferred forward.
e)   With the torso thrown forward, the HEAD is thrown back so that the face looks up.
f)   ELBOWS are sharply pulled back as the torso is thrust forward, causing the forearms to move back also.

FIGURE 22a

Position

a & b)   As for Figure 22.
c)   The PELVIS is curved forward with a slight scoop in the upper region.
d)   The stomach contracts so that the upper body is scooped in. The TORSO is thus curved towards the back.
e)   The HEAD completes the scoop started in the pelvis by dropping forward.
f)   The ARMS are positioned as for Figure 22 except that the elbows are pushed forward. The hands go towards the centre.

Motion

a & b)   As for Figure 22 Motion.
c)   The PELVIS is pushed forward, the ishium leading. The illium scoops in as the stomach contracts.
d)   The TORSO curves inward in one sharp motion as the weight is transferred.
e)   The HEAD falls forward with the curve of the torso.
f)   From being pulled back, the ELBOWS are pushed forward, the hands moving towards the centre.

Figures 22 and 22a together form one Revival motion. They are repeated alternately numerous times. The breath is heavily exhaled with Figure 22 as the torso is arched forward, and inhaled with Figure 22a.

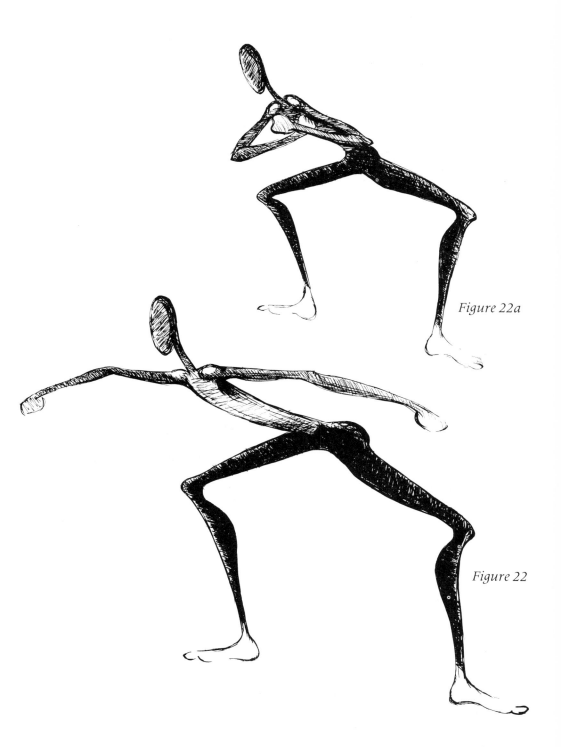

Figure 22a

Figure 22

81

FIGURE 23: 'The Bell Ringer'

Position

a) The FEET are placed flat on the floor in second position (feet about 12″ apart).
b) The KNEES are slightly bent but the body retains an upward lift.
c) The body retains its natural relationship to the knees and torso.
d) The TORSO is lifted up slightly as the stomach muscles are tightened.
e) The HEAD lifts back to look diagonally upward, shaking slightly.
f) The ARMS are stretched above the head. The hands are clasped together slightly forward on the head.

Position 23a

a) Both FEET are in second position flat on the floor.
b) The KNEES bend.
c) The PELVIS is dropped in line with the thighs.
d) The TORSO is curved over slightly forward between the knees.
e) The HEAD looks down.
f) The ARMS, hands clasped together, are held down between the knees. The elbows bend slightly.

Motion

Figures 23 & 23a

a) The dancer performs a quick *small* jump, landing on one foot before the other. The FEET remain in place as he moves into position 23a.
b) As the dancer jumps, the KNEES remain straight. When the feet touch the floor the knees bend deeper and deeper to arrive at figure 23a where the knees are fully bent and the dancer is low to the ground.
c) The PELVIS is shaken quickly side to side as the knees bend.
d) The TORSO is also rapidly shaken laterally as the knees bend, stopping only when the knees are fully bent. The torso bends slightly forward at this point.
e) The HEAD looks down gradually as the body lowers.
f) From being held up above the head, the elbows are bent and the ARMS are pulled down in front of the body, shaking vigorously from side to side as the torso shakes. The hands are held together – the movement is called the 'Bell Ringer' – and the dancer, holding the 'bell' in both hands, rings it by shaking it down in front of the body.

FIGURE 24

Position

a) Both FEET are placed in second position, casually turned out.
b) The KNEES are bent in line with the feet.
c) The PELVIS is dropped or relaxed in its natural relation to other body parts.

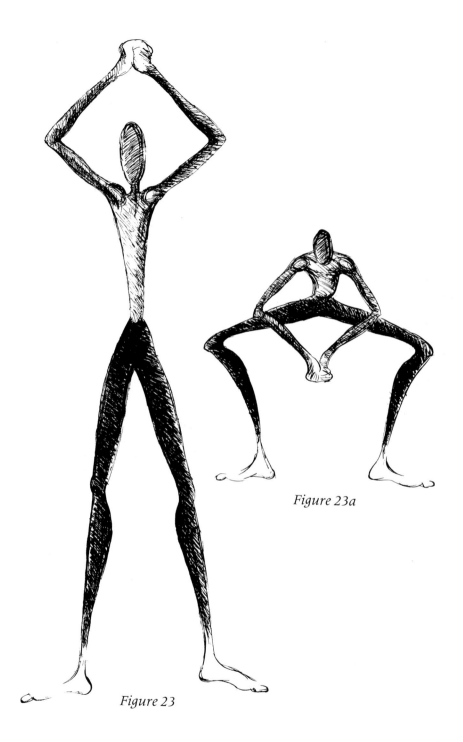

Figure 23a

Figure 23

d) The TORSO is pitched slightly forward. The natural curve in the back is kept.
e) The HEAD is lifted and may be thrown back with the chin jutting forward.
f) The right ARM is lifted above the head. The elbow is bent slightly so that the line is broken. The fingers are relaxed or held in a relaxed fist. The left arm reflects the right but is held down towards the knees.

Motion

a) The FEET remain on the floor.
b) The KNEES bounce, taking the weight of the body up and down on a regular 4/4 beat. The body can be kept central or transferred laterally from side to side as the dancer moves.
c) The PELVIS reflects the bounce in the knees.
d) The ribcage is pushed out and pulled back in a movement which basically exaggerates the natural breath patterns. This is also on a 4/4 beat.
e) The HEAD is rhythmically thrown back with the bounce of the body.
f) The ARMS, remaining relaxed, are lifted and dropped alternately as the body bounces. The movement may be small so that the wrists reach shoulder level or this may be further exaggerated so that they reach above the head with each lift.

Variations on Basic Positions and Motions

As with all folk dances, variation through improvisation plays a great role in Revival. Each participant uses the movements shown, not as acts of worship in themselves but as a medium through which to reach God. The movements are, for the most part, simple and repetitive and it is through the individual movements of the participants, as they reach various levels of trance, that variation occurs.

One basic variation throughout Revival is the use of vibration. The participant will, at random, shake all or some body parts, emphasising the fervour of the moment. This shaking may build up until, in 'Myal' the dancer will drop to the floor while continuing to shake (see Possession above).

Figure 19
The dancer may take two small steps forward on the right foot, accompanied by a double hunch forward of the shoulders and torso in double tempo. The left foot still takes one step to join the right.

Figure 21
This motion can be completed with the dancer simply transferring the weight from one foot to the other so that the feet hardly leave the floor. If the tempo of the song is slow, however, the dancer will tilt far over to the left side, allowing the right foot to extend onto the toes or just off the floor.

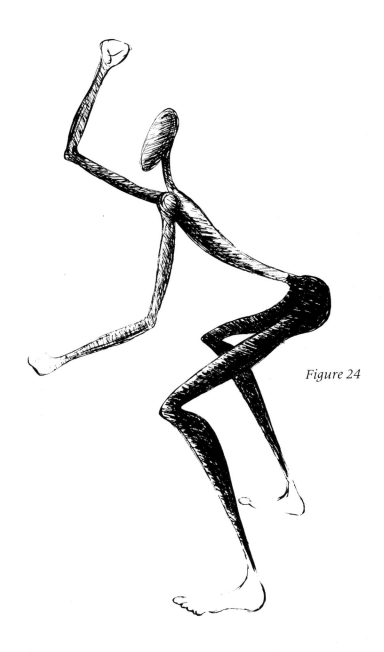

Figure 24

1. Apart from Barbados and Antigua, no other islands have been so consistently influenced by Britain.
2. Smith (1980), p. iv.
3. Smith (1980), p. 13.
4. Smith, 'Bruckin's', Jamaica School of Dance (1980).
5. Pocomania is now more frequently and correctly referred to as 'Pukkumina', thus establishing a link with Kumina and Myal, rather than the translation 'pocomania' (a little madness) given it by the unsympathetic onlookers who first wrote about it.
6. *The Musical Quarterly*, Vol. 16 (1930), from Patterson (1973), p. 212.
7. Hence the Zionists stop at the number 60 when 'Trumping' (see 'The Ritual of Revival', pp. 67–70), while the Pocomania sect continue to 61, further into Africanism.
8. Patterson (1973), p. 215.
9. Seaga, 'Revival Cults in Jamaica', *Jamaica Journal*, Vol. 3 No. 2 (1969).
10. Baxter (1970), p. 142.
11. Also referred to as 'Labouring'. Seaga (1969), p. 79.
12. Seaga, *op. cit.*, p.7.
13. *Ibid.*

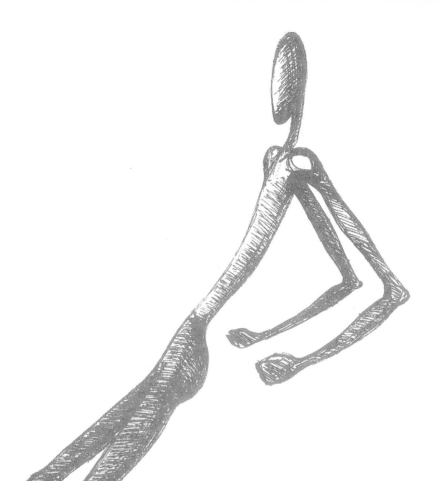

CHAPTER FOUR

Commonalities Between the Folk Dances of Jamaica: The Jamaican Folk Technique

Abstraction: Towards a Technique

Commonalities Between the Folk Dances of Jamaica: The Jamaican Folk Technique

The Jamaican folk technique is an assimilation of the main principles and elements evident within the different Jamaican folk dances. These principles are sifted out to find the common ground between the dances and from here a general technique can be developed. The Jamaican technique is, necessarily, representative of the Caribbean folk technique. Most Caribbean islands share the same basic history; that of invasion, occupation and domination by alien cultures. Thus, characteristics and principles that have evolved in the formation of the Jamaican technique contributed also to the Caribbean technique as a whole. Among these principles are the following:

• One of the first principles of the technique is that of earth-bound movement and the maintenance of a low centre of gravity. In Kumina and Dinkie Minie in particular and, to some extent, in Bruckin's and the Camp Style Quadrille, the bodies are bent low to the ground. This is an African retention.

• The feet are usually flat on the floor and elevation, a European trait more evident in the Ballroom Style Quadrille, is minimal.

• Much use is made of the flexed foot – in Dinkie Minie with the *heel* lifted, Bruckin's with the *toe* lifted, and in the breaks from the Camp Style Quadrille.

• Much Caribbean movement is centred around the pelvis, particularly in dances revealing more African retentions, such as Dinkie Minie (where the forces of procreation are flaunted in defiance of death), Kumina, Bruckin's and the Mento figure of the Camp Style Quadrille. The hips and pelvis must be relaxed and free to swing independently.

• Arms are predominantly bent, even if the flexion is slight. It is unusual to see a straight arm in Jamaican folk dance (except, perhaps, in cases like Revival, where the upward mobility of the prayers to the Heavenly Spirits encourage arms to be lifted high into the air). Whether close to the side in basket-holding position, carried forward, akimbo (on hips) or pushed back, the elbows will be bent. This is in keeping with the characteristic of broken lines in the African-derived Caribbean technique. Arms may be functional, carrying objects such as rum, goat, plates of food (Kumina, Dinkie Minie), fans (Quadrille), or swords (Bruckin's).

• The face of the Jamaican dancer retains a 'cool' expression. Even while performing suggestive movements, mourning the death of a loved one or celebrating a marriage or birth, the face remains calm with a relaxed aura. The *body* is expressive in gesture.

• Isolations are another basic feature of Jamaican folk dance. Often the body parts will work alone: the shoulders, pelvis, feet, hands will often move independently of the accompanying body parts to complete the movement. This is done for emphasis or design and is clearly evident in Bruckin's (see Variations on Basic Positions and Motions).

• Polyrhythms are a basic feature of African dance and music. Musically, this involves a number of different rhythms being played simultaneously to complete the tune heard. In dance terms this involves different parts of the body moving in different rhythms, e.g. the feet following a basic 4/4 pattern while the torso picks up on the 2/4 beat. This is well exemplified in Kumina, where Professor Rex Nettleford has pin-pointed the motion of the arms swinging across the body in 6/8 time, while the pelvis and feet pick up the basic 2/4 of the Kbandu (bass drum).[1]

Abstraction: Towards a Technique

For a very long time, Jamaican folk dances have been used 'as is' – in their raw form – to celebrate births, marriages, deaths, social or religious occurrences. They have, for the most part, remained in their natural environments, so much so that it is rare to see Bruckin's performed outside Portland, or Dinkie Minie outside St Mary or Kingston. Today, however, more and more educators and choreographers are beginning to realise the value of folk dances within the school time-table and as a source for creative dancing. On the educational side, it is all too often proven that the children with an active interest in dance learn to apply the discipline of that medium to their other school subjects. The desire to look good and perform well becomes part of the child's personality and goals. At Jessie Rippol and St Aloysius schools in Kingston for example, dance tutors Patricia Noble and Pauline Power respectively, have an excellent record of disciplined students and passes in the Common Entrance Examination. If properly applied, Jamaican folk dances can be used to assist other subjects such as history. The Quadrille provides an excellent guideline to the European court society while Kumina, with its use of ancestor worship through dance and song, can aid the teaching of African life and history. Revival, with its unique blend of Myal and Christian religions, can be used to draw out the similarities of worship between alien civilisations etc. The use of dance as an aid to teaching reveals a fresh approach to education very often needed to gain and keep the attention of today's child.

In their raw form, the folk dances need no additions to justify their value and use as recreational, educational and religious stimulants. Over the years they have evolved and developed within a natural process of environmental and social change and, if given scope, will continue to do so as an intrinsic part of Jamaican life. For the student of dance, however, the Jamaican folk dances can provide a rich and staple diet from which to gain inspiration for new ideas and movements. It is at this area which we now look.

Abstraction is the process of using material drawn from life as a source for new development; 'withdrawal; stealing; elimination of the concrete' (Oxford Dictionary). Emphasis is placed on the word 'concrete', indicating that abstraction deals with the established basics of the subject matter and not its embellishments. Professor Nettleford cites the need for defining the *core* of the subject, what he terms the 'irreducible kernel', before one begins to abstract, so as to avoid the vagueness of working with idiocyncrasies and the peripheries of the subject matter. In general terms the actual process of abstraction can be carried out in a number of ways. What is important is the development of the original in the creation of the new. These developments may include:

a) Variation of movement, i.e. making it smaller or larger.
b) Use of contrasting movements, i.e. juxtaposing slow tempo movements with quick tempo ones.

c) Variation of rhythm, i.e. breaking up the basic rhythm pattern to create new phrases.

d) Variation in the use of space, levels, i.e. high, medium and low.

e) Variation in flow, i.e. movement quality.

More specifically, the method of 'Motif Development' can be used. In the dance context, four stages are evident:

1. Decide on the original, i.e. the motif. This may be one movement or a number of movements linked together.

2. Look at the specifics of the movement(s) in terms of the positioning and motions of the feet, pelvis, torso, arms, head, etc.

3. Develop or extend these one by one to create a new movement, making sure that the link with the source is still evident. The most obvious means of development is through enlargement. Here a slight arm or leg movement can become a grand sweeping movement or step. Other means of development include variation on the accent or dynamics of the movement; on the quality – from sharp and percussive to smooth and continuous; on the level of the movement – a walk may be taken into a hop or jump into the air, or an arm movement performed standing up in the original may be repeated in a kneeling position in the development.

4. After this development stage has been repeated a number of times, using a variety of motifs taken from the same source, the student will become familiar with the *essence* of the subject rather than the specifics. For example, when a number of motifs have been found and experimented upon, the dancer will begin to see a consistency of elements, e.g. bent elbows and knees, flat back pitched forward, use of flexed feet etc, and will recognise these as the 'irreducible kernel' of the folk form.

This process can be further clarified using one of the Jamaican folk dances as source: Bruckin's.

1. The chosen motif is Bruckin's Figure 15.

2. The specifics of the movement include:
    a) the diagonal tilt of the body;
    b) the bent arm held in at the sides;
    c) the pelvis pushed forward;
    d) the use of a flexed foot.

3. a) Diagonals may be varied through degrees of tilt; the tilt may be performed sideways laterally; it may be taken into off-balance and this too can vary in degrees.

    b) The small circular pathway of the arm may be extended and the arm fully outstretched before it is brought in to the sides.

    c) The forward push of the pelvis may be developed through use of dynamics. Rather than pushing the pelvis forward at the regular tempo, the push may be percussively accentuated in one instance and smoothly carried forward in another.

    d) In Figure 15 the heel of the flexed foot remains on the floor. In developing this aspect, the heel could be lifted off the floor, the foot pointed temporarily before being flexed again and then placed to the side or back.

4. If the student then uses the other figures of Bruckin's as source he will eventually reduce the essence of Bruckin's down to a small number of elements: the tilt of the body; the push forward of the pelvis; the jerk or snap of the torso; the flexed foot etc. Consideration must also be given to the particular accent of the Bruckin's movement, which is percussive. Having established the elements, the student should then try to choreograph a small movement sequence based not on Bruckin's the original but the *elements* of Bruckin's. The second level of abstraction is thus begun and if this process is repeated with other Jamaican folk dance forms one may begin to abstract from the Jamaican folk dance as a single entity. From *this* source a technique based on the Jamaican folk forms can be created.

    Technical abstraction, however – i.e. abstraction from the basic movements of the folk form – is not enough, states Professor Nettleford.[2] One must have a knowledge of the background to the form – its origins, usage and characteristics – so as to facilitate an abstraction from those elements also. All aspects of the dance form must eventually be studied before the true abstraction will be arrived at.

1. Professor Rex Nettleford, 'Kumina', Jamaica School of Dance (May 1984).
2. 'Abstraction of Traditional Folk Forms', Jamaica School of Dance (May 1984).

Conclusion

The folk dances of Jamaica, it has been shown, have evolved directly out of the history of its people. Without the Spanish and British invasions the country might have remained in the hands of the Arawaks, causing a completely different historical evolution. Without the introduction of the sugar plantations, the racial breakdown of the Jamaican population would most likely be different. Things indigenous to Jamaica, such as the folk dances discussed, most often reveal a blending of African and British, from time to time tempered with a measure of Indian or Chinese culture. The task now at hand is to place the Jamaican folk dances in the context of Jamaica today: just where do the folk dances fit into Jamaican society, if indeed they fit in at all?

The histories given have indicated a certain regional exclusiveness to each folk form and, unfortunately, this exclusiveness is still prevalent today: if one wishes to see a Kumina ceremony, one has to visit St Thomas; Bruckin's is virtually extinct except in Portland; and the Quadrille as a social dance is rarely seen. Dinkie Minie, very much alive in St Mary, is scarcely performed in the other parishes (apart from Hanover and West Moreland where its sister form Gerreh exists). Of all the folk dances dealt with, Revival is the most widely used as Revival bands from either Pocomania or Zionist cults can be found in each parish. It is highly probable, therefore, that in the future an indigenous form like Bruckin's may well be forgotten by the majority of Jamaicans. Indeed, it is mainly through the work of pioneers like Ivy Baxter and Professor Rex Nettleford, along with the work of the Cultural Development Commission, that they are known at all. The Festival of Arts, a yearly event run by the Jamaican Cultural Development Commission, offers the greatest single outlet for folk dance exposure. Participants, from children to adults, are encouraged to display their particular skills in all art forms. It is here that the majority of folk dances can be seen, as groups vie for awards of excellence. The importance of the Festival cannot be over-stressed, as it offers a chance for the whole of Jamaica to view the art forms, either at the Festival itself or on television. Even more important, the Festival's policy of parish workshops going into schools and community centres ensures the teaching of these forms to children, and hence ensures some future for the Jamaican art forms. Understandably, the Festival of Arts, which climaxes in July and August each year, is a major event on the Jamaican calendar.

With the Festival of Arts taking place annually, it might be fair to assume a general knowledge and value of the Jamaican folk forms amongst the majority of people. However, for dance in particular, this is not the case. As with most folk culture, the traditonal folk dances of Jamaica are to be found not only in specific areas but also amongst the lower classes of society, where, it is stated, people stick closer to their roots.[1] Amongst the middle and upper classes, less, if any, such culture is actually practised and exposure is mainly through the television. Throughout Jamaica, however, there is often a negative attitude toward Jamaican art and things Jamaican in general. A trait of colonisation:

> Deeper than the political forms of colonisation went the mentality it imposed on a subject population and Jamaica has hardly begun to free herself from this inheritance; from the habit of trying, however unsuccessfully, to look at the world through British eyes.[2]

Not only the world but Jamaica itself is looked at through foreign eyes and, not surprisingly therefore, the folk culture is derogatively viewed and its place in society is an increasingly precarious one. While thousands of tourists visit the country and revel in the folk dances they see, the majority of Jamaicans merely 'tolerate' these while embracing the latest trends from outside the Caribbean. Cheryl Ryman writes in *Jamaica Journal*:

> At all levels of society we need to reassess our attitudes to the agents of our heritage. The tendency to consider and treat many of our traditional forms (primarily of African origin) carelessly and with a display of 'foreign' ignorance, is all too prevalent . . . A population that is some 90% African in origin, carries a deeply conditioned negative African-Caribbean self-image, while aspiring to an ultimately unattainable Euro-centric ideal. This schizoid situation not only persists but forms a significant part of our explosive reality. Anything therefore which contributes to the continuation of this schizophrenia is self-damaging . . . this is one legacy of the colonial experience which must be shed.[3]

For many years now writers and critics alike have pin-pointed this remnant of colonisation as a major contributor to the negative attitude towards Jamaican art. Still, this attitude persists. In this negative action, the 'people' – i.e. the majority – perhaps follow the example set by the agents of control – the government, community leaders, educational establishments etc. – who, by themselves looking outward for set values, indicate a greater respect for alien cultures and ideals. The apparent strength of America, whose society Jamaica strives to emulate, is that facets of *American* history and culture are being used to teach their children and build their nation. Surely it would be more profitable to emulate *this* American example: to focus on the history and culture that is indigenous to Jamaica and, by defining its characteristic features, strengths and weaknesses, morals and values, develop criteria for education and nation building – *Jamaican* nation building. Only then will things Jamaican be given their full value.

1. Perhaps because their levels of exposure (through travel for instance) and hence their levels of influence, is often limited.
2. Norris (1962), p. 71.
3. Number 44, p. 3.